the multifacial make-up book

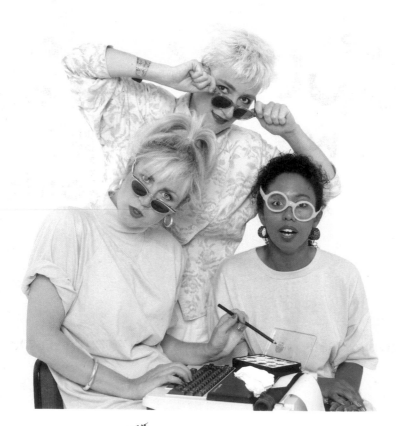

photography
by
Corinne
Turner

the multifacial make-up book

A PRACTICAL GUIDE

by

Sarah Greene, Vicky Licorish and Wendy Freeman

BLOOMSBURY

First published in Great Britain 1987

Bloomsbury Publishing Ltd, 2 Soho Square, London W1

British Library Cataloguing in Publication Data

Greene. Sarah
  The multifacial make-up book: a practical guide
1. Cosmetics   2. Face – care and hygiene
I. Title   II. Licorish, Vicky
III. Freeman, Wendy
646.7′26′088042 RA778

ISBN 0 7475 0100 9

Designed by Barbon Communications Ltd
2 Barbon Close London WC1N 3JX

Art Director: Sue Rawkins

Designer: Chris Sessions

Illustrations: Wendy Freeman and Chris Sessions

Phototypeset: Chapterhouse, The Cloisters, Formby, L37 3PX

Printed in Italy

contents

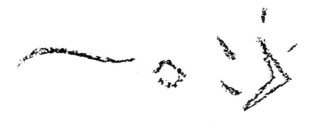

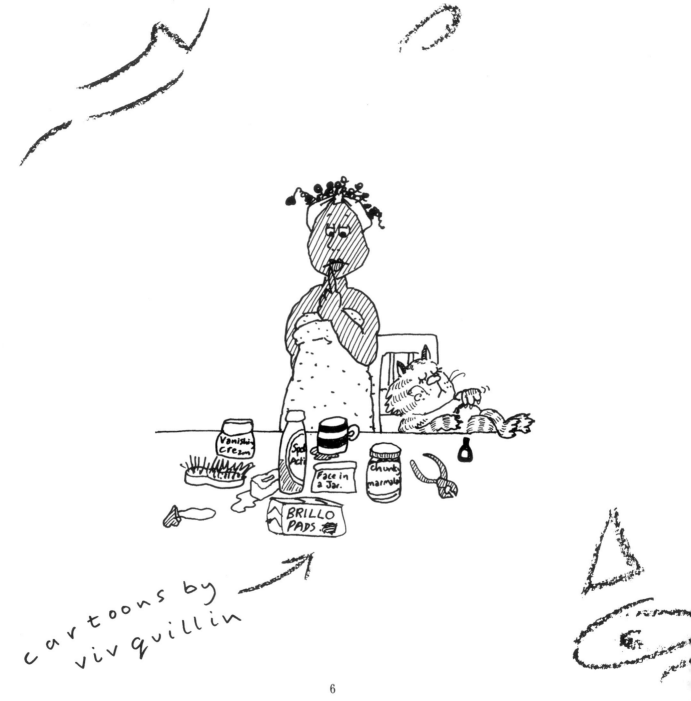

cartoons by
viv quillin

basics

Treat this book as a manual. We hope it will inform, suggest and entertain, rather than preach or lay down the law... how CAN you make hard and fast rules about make-up, when every face is so completely different? Of course, whilst we acknowledge that each skin type, colour, texture and shape has its own specific needs, it's only by *swapping* ideas and 'secrets' that you can begin to create your very own look and have some fun.

The next bit of the book is a questionnaire. Have a good think before you fill it in. It's only you who'll see the answers, so be really honest with yourself! Hopefully by the end of it you'll have built up a picture of what your own personal needs are. After all, the more your make-up complements your personality and style, the better it will look and feel.

When you've filled in the questionnaire, keep that image of yourself in your mind as you read the book, and as you look at the skin-tone chart.

Find the nearest colours to your own skin and use the corresponding numbers for reference later. The range of colours may surprise you – but that's deliberate. If you have a dark skin you'll be only too familiar with the blank stares of cosmetics salesladies who just can't understand your reluctance to buy the last remaining bottle of '*Washed-Out Peach*' on offer. Similarly, if you're fair-skinned, ever tried making '*Barely-Alive*' look like it's your own?! The 'Where to Find It' section at the back of the book should be of some help here. Let's face it, one person's skin tone can alter throughout the month, let alone the year, so you may find you cross over several different tones.

By the way... two more things before you start: a) We'd like you to look like YOU – *not* a fashion victim!... and b) You don't *have* to wear any make-up at all... but if you *do* fancy having some fun experimenting – grab hold of a mirror and...

read on for 'who are you?'

questionnaire

Look in the mirror – what do you see?

What colour is your hair? _____

What about your eyes? _____

What colour are they? _____

What shape are they? _____

Do you wear contact lenses or glasses? _____

Your skin: what type is it? _____ What condition is it in? _____

What shape is your face? _____

Which feature do you like best? _____

What do you dislike most about your face? _____

How old are you? _____

Are you an extrovert or an introvert? _____

How do you spend most of your time? _____

Where do you spend most of your time? _____

Do you think about what you eat? _____

Do you smoke? _____

Do you drink alcohol?

Do you exercise?

How much sleep do you get?

Do you wear make-up?

If 'no', why not?

If 'yes', why?

How long does it take you to put it on?

Do you take it off every night?

Do you wear it all day? Or just on certain occasions?

List the items of make-up you use regularly.

How much do you spend on make-up?

List the skin care items you use regularly
and how much you spend on them.

How happy do you feel about the way you look?

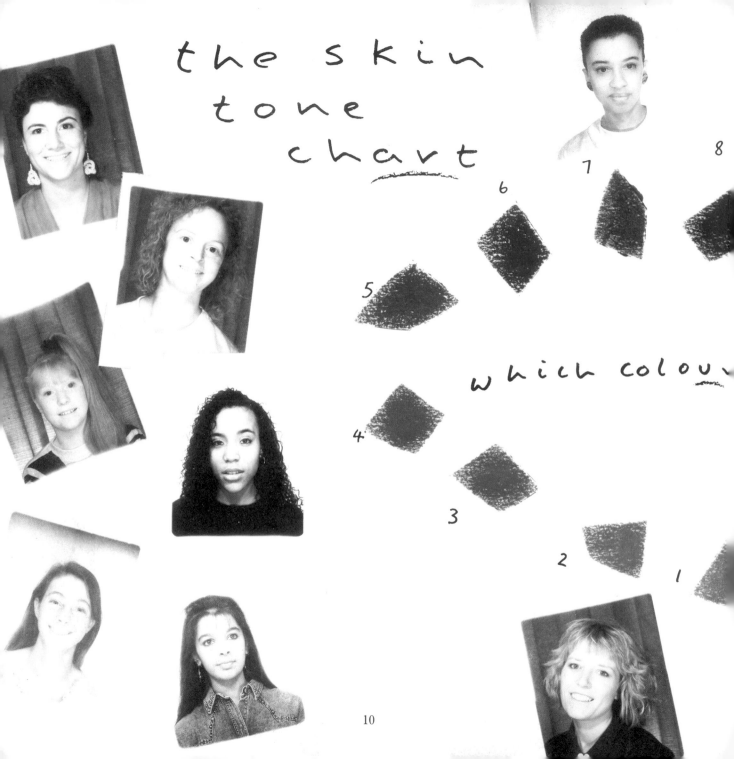

the skin tone chart

which colou

8

7

6

5

4

3

2

1

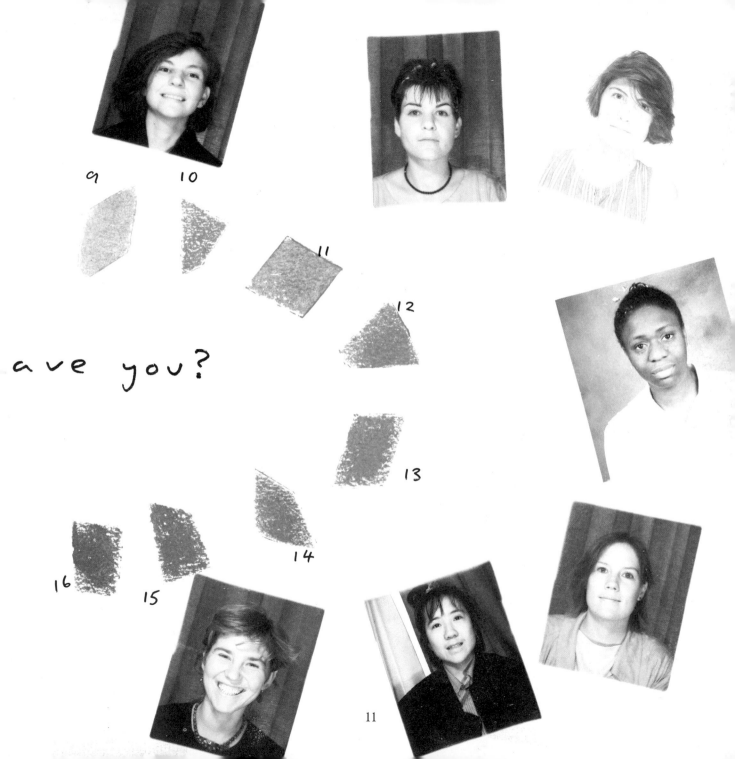

9 10

11

12

ave you?

13

14

16 15

11

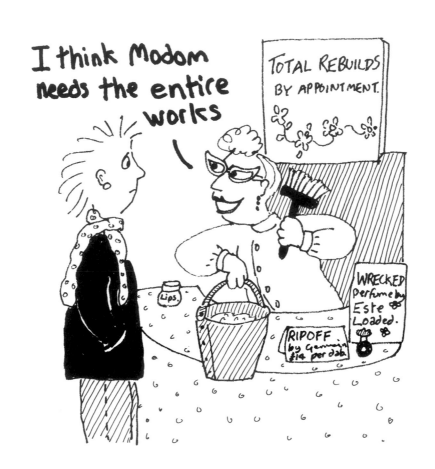

buying and applying

- make-up bags
- foundation
- camouflage
- sculpting
- eyes
- lipstick
- hands and nails

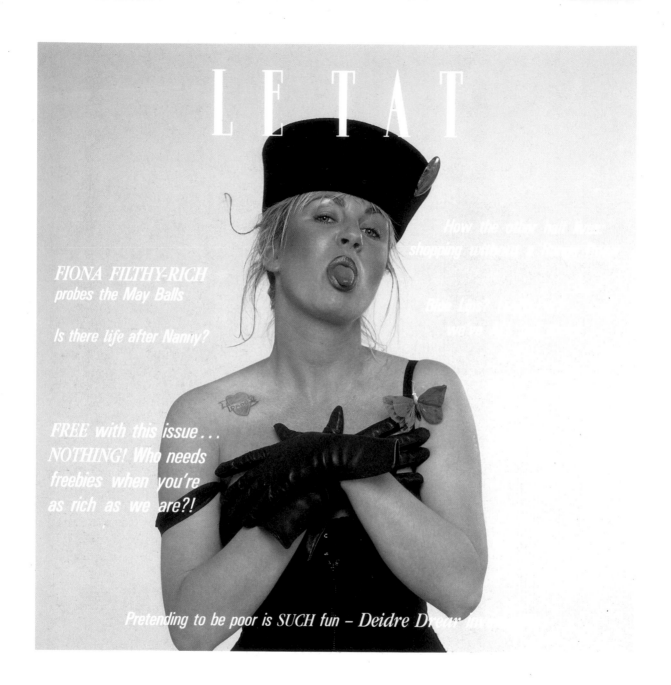

LE TAT

FIONA FILTHY-RICH
probes the May Balls

Is there life after Nanny?

FREE with this issue . . .
NOTHING! Who needs
freebies when you're
as rich as we are?!

How the other half live:
shopping without a care

Boo Gili

Pretending to be poor is SUCH fun – Deidre Dream in

14

COSMIC

IVORY BONES talks frankly
about her naughty
nips and tucks...

How to make-up
for your man!!!

GOLD! GOLD! GOLD!
is there any other colour, girls?

Knit your own false eyelashes
– free pattern inside...

How to be a sex goddess
– Spangley Tips reveals her
beauty secrets!!

FREE INSIDE –
DIY nose job kit! /
Ivory Bones' nips and tucks

COMPETITION! Gums are back in fashion – Win £6,000
worth of cosmetic dentistry

Your buying

Make-up is BIG BUSINESS.

Fact: we spend £212,000,000 a year on make-up.

The cosmetics industry depends on consumers like you and me for its very survival. It creates needs and problems we never knew we had, and the products to solve them. To get us to part with our money it uses glossy and expensive adverts, the cost of which is ultimately added to the price we pay in the shops. It's a vicious circle. So, don't be fooled into paying massive prices because of a high-profile advertising campaign or, more importantly, glamorous packaging. Watch out for gimmicks and fads.

The woman working on the make-up counter is there to help you and it's worth remembering that. But she is also on the front line of the industry, she is helping to keep its huge wheels turning and must therefore achieve target sales every week. Incentive schemes and bonuses will continually encourage her to sell, sell, sell, and you to buy. A good saleswoman isn't going to let you get

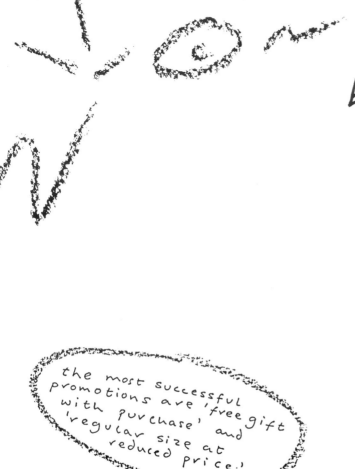

the most successful promotions are 'free gift with purchase' and 'regular size at reduced price.'

away with buying one mascara when she could be selling you the whole range... even if it takes a freebie to tempt you! So, whilst making use of all the testers and the assistant's genuine expertise, stick to your guns (and your wallet!) and don't be intimidated.

Ever considered why you're standing at the make-up counter in the first place? It could have something to do with that spangly picture you saw in a magazine. Chances are you don't look very like the model in the picture... but then, neither does she in real life. She only looked like that the moment the photograph was taken. When, at long last the photographer had managed to get the perfect shot, the model gave the clothes back to the designer, the jewels and the car back to the stylist and the boyfriend back to the model agency. The make-up artist wiped off the hours of work, the hairdresser combed out layers of lacquer and mousse and the photographer's assistant switched off the lights.

We're not saying 'don't buy make-up' – we're just saying don't be conned...

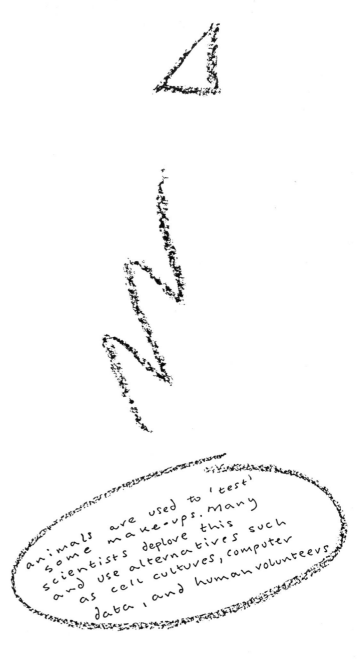

animals are used to 'test' some make-ups. many scientists deplore this and use alternatives such as cell cultures, computer data, and human volunteers

a ~ pencil
     sharpener
with two size holes

b ~ powder
     brush

c ~ sponge
   –essential for
    applying foundation

d ~ blusher brush

e ~ chisel ended
        tweezers

f ~ eyebrow brush
     and comb

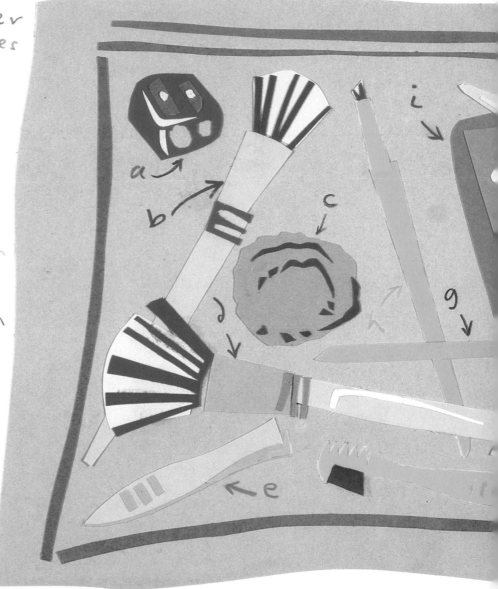

tissues and cotton wool are al
  essentials for the complete
18

g

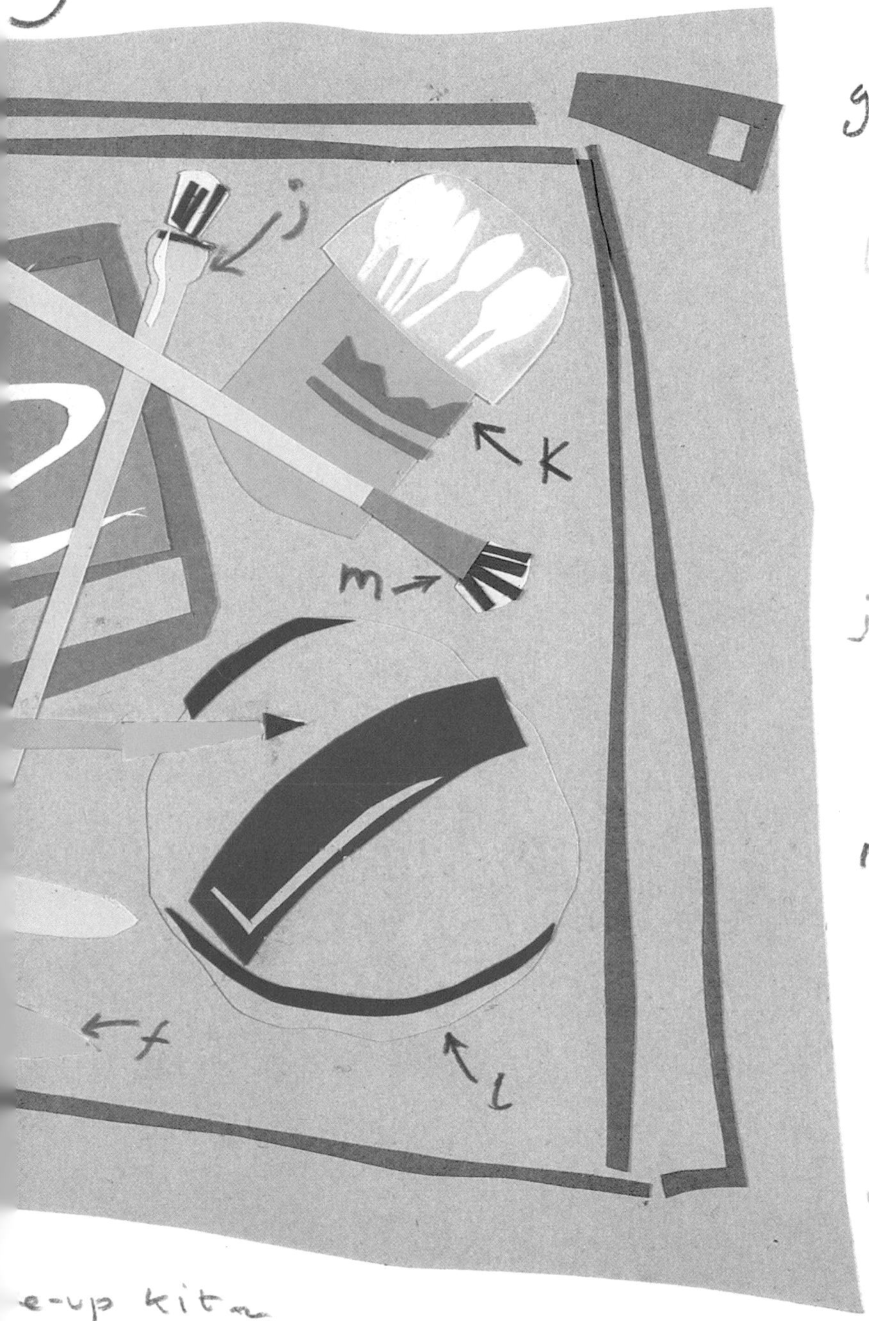

g ~ thin brush

h ~ lip brush

i magnifying mirror

j ~ chisel ended brush
for eyeshadows
and blending

K ~ cotton wool buds

L ~ powder puff
buy a good old
fashioned velour
one

m ~ broad brush
for foundation
+ eyeshadows

e-up kit ~

zapps

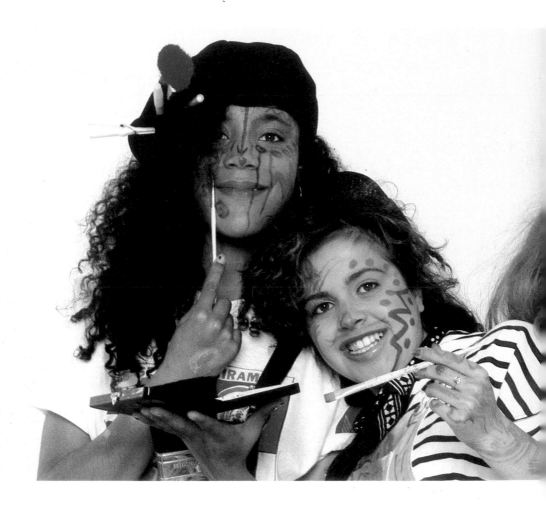

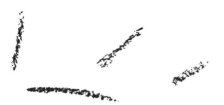

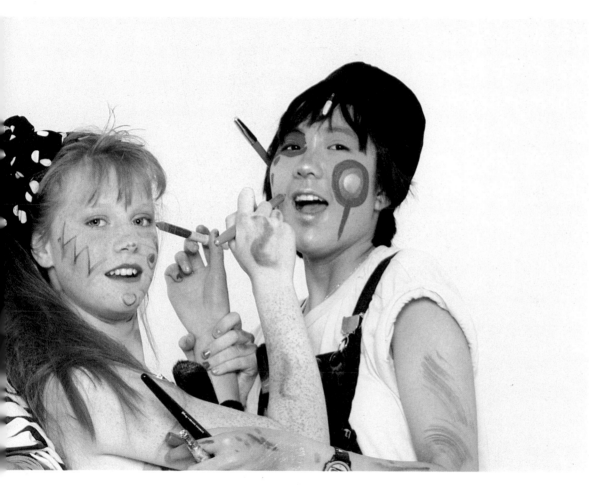

POW

am

confused?.. read on

foundation

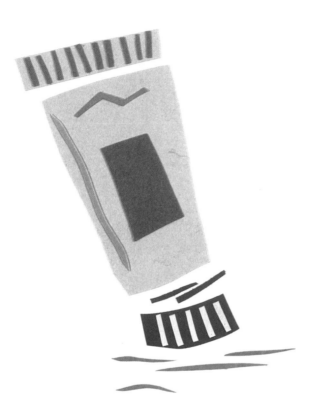

The main reasons for using foundation or 'base' are to even out your natural skin tone and cover light blemishes. It's probably the most basic raw material you'll need, so take plenty of time to find exactly the right one for you. Here are a few shopping tips:

Arm yourself with a small mirror, a packet of tissues, a good, truthful friend and a confident attitude. Set off with *no* make-up on . . .

It helps if you can get to a department store or a well-stocked chain-store, where there should be a good selection of cosmetics in all price ranges. In fact, the *apparent* range of bottles, tubes and charts can look very bewildering – so where do you start?

There are four main types of foundation: *liquid*, *cream*, *cake* and *tint*.

LIQUID and CREAM foundations can be suitable for both oily and dry skins, so look for a base with added moisturiser if you have a dry skin, or for one termed 'oil-free' or 'water-based' if your skin is oily.

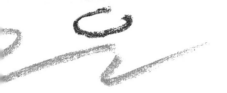

CAKE foundation is thick and dry in consistency giving a flatter, more 'matt' look – also good for oily skins.

TINTS or GELS are the most transparent of all – great for a 'no make-up' or tanned look. Some even contain a sunscreen to protect your skin.

The names of these four main types of base vary from brand to brand, but they generally refer to the consistency of the product. To get an idea of the effect a foundation will have (over your whole face – rather than just a small blob!) a good rule of thumb is: the runnier it is, the lighter or thinner the coverage. If you're unsure about the consistency of the tester you want to try, read the blurb on the bottle or ask the assistant. By the way, check with the 'skin care' section if you're not sure about what type of skin you have. But if you know you have sensitive skin, try to find a suitable base which has been labelled 'hypo-allergenic' – it'll be less likely to cause an allergic reaction than competing brands.

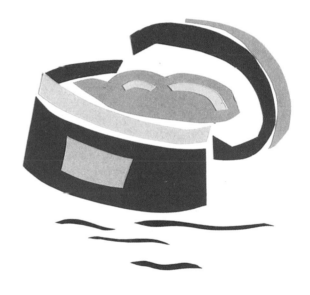

now for colour

colour

Feel free to try out as many testers as you want: test on your face and not your hand, as the two types of skin are rarely the same colour (this is where the tissues come in useful!!). Dab on a small blob and smooth it in. If it appears to blend in with your own skin tone, then it's the right one for you.

Now this may sound quick and easy in theory, but in practice it may take a long time and many different blobs of colour before you're completely satisfied. Your skin tone may fall *between* two different bases so, especially with the cheaper ranges, consider buying two and mixing them. This is also useful for the times when your skin tone changes slightly (after hols and so on).

If at all possible, check the colour in daylight, with your mirror in hand and your friend in tow. Let the assistant know and don't forget to leave the tester itself behind – you don't want to get carted off for shoplifting! This may all seem like a bit of a palaver, but artificial lighting can be very deceptive. All your hard work will be worth it in the end because, with any luck, you'll only have to do it once.

This will come as good news to you if you have a dark skin because, although the situation is improving gradually, there is still a ridiculously small range of colours for you to choose from. Hopefully, the 'Where to find it' section (page 85) will point you in the right direction for stockists.

Another handy hint is to get friendly with the saleslady, who may have all sorts of useful information and brand names tucked away. As we said earlier, she *is* there to help you, so, whatever colour you are it might be fun to ask her to apply your base for you. But, establish first that it's her *advice* you're after, not necessarily the product – that way you don't feel pressured and your friend can justify her or his presence by handing out moral support and tissues to wipe off what you don't like!

don't try to hide freckles with this foundation ~ they're pretty

24

powder

Lots of people can't be bothered with powder because they think of it as old fashioned, something their grandmas used to wear. In fact, it is essential for 'fixing' your make-up and making it last longer.

You can buy powder in two forms: *loose* or *compact*. Loose powder is very fine, so it can be very messy to carry around . . . but, as it's really the best type for fixing, use it at home and leave it there. Compacts are portable and great for quick re-touching jobs.

Powder itself can be *translucent* (transparent), *coloured* or *iridescent* (sparkly). Try to find a truly translucent powder as then it won't change the colour of your foundation. Obviously, it's a good idea to buy your powder at the same time as your base – to test how well they match. Coloured powders give a denser finish and must match your foundation exactly. Iridescent powder is great for parties and for a sparkly dramatic look . . . but . . . WARNING! . . . For that really sweaty look, put it on all over your face!! Seriously, use iridescent very sparingly for the bits you want to highlight. See the 'Sculpting' section for further tips (page 32).

ANOTHER WARNING!! . . . If you keep re-applying powder from a compact, it can go very 'cakey' – so go easy.

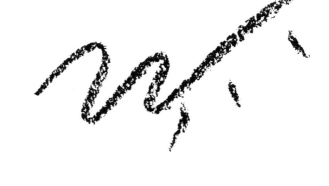

coming next~
applying foundation
and powder

applying foundation

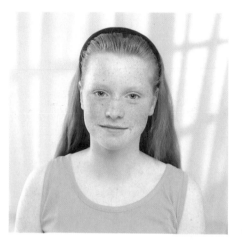
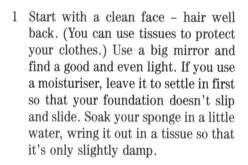

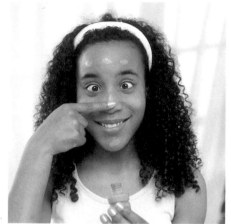
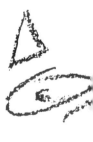
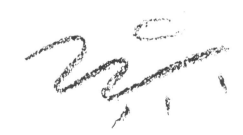

1 Start with a clean face – hair well back. (You can use tissues to protect your clothes.) Use a big mirror and find a good and even light. If you use a moisturiser, leave it to settle in first so that your foundation doesn't slip and slide. Soak your sponge in a little water, wring it out in a tissue so that it's only slightly damp.

2 Blob your foundation onto your forehead, cheeks, nose, chin and neck.

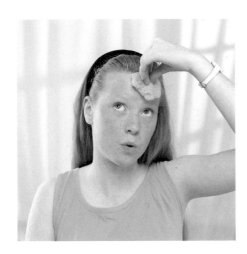 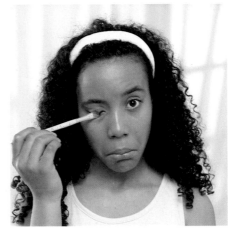

3 Using the sponge, smooth it over your face from the centre outwards so that you're not left with a heavy outline around the edge of your face, neck and hairline.

4 Don't forget the nooks and crannies! Particularly round your nose, under your eyes and over your eyelids.

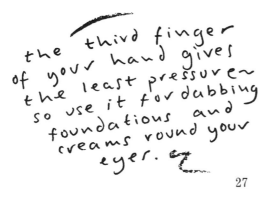

the third finger of your hand gives the least pressure~ so use it for dabbing foundations and creams round your eyes. ~

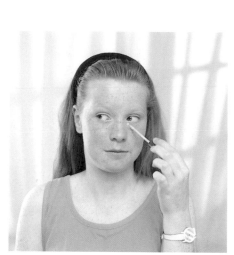

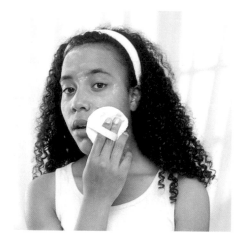

5 If you need to use a concealer to cover any blemishes, this is the time to do it. Dot it on the areas you want to conceal and smooth it out so that it blends in with your foundation. (See over the page for the more serious 'Camouflage' techniques.)

6 Powder next – dip the puff into the powder and pat it generously over your face. Take care not to rub as this will smear your foundation.

watch out for foundation & powder sticking to your eyelashes – brush it away using an eyelash brush.

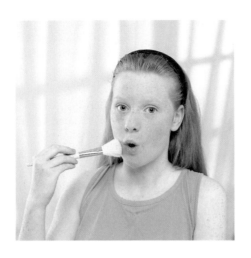

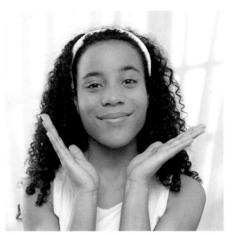

7 Brush off the excess powder with a big fat brush for...

8 The finished look!

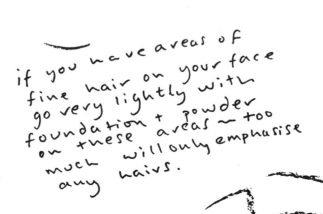

if you have areas of fine hair on your face go very lightly with foundation + powder on these areas ~ too much will only emphasise any hairs.

camouflage

Zits, bags, wrinkles, birthmarks, scars and broken veins . . . take the paper bag off your head and take heart – help is close at hand.

Any disfigurement can seriously affect your confidence and the way you feel about the world. Never be tempted to pile on layers of your usual foundation to cover up one of the types of problems listed above. There is a variety of amazing, specially-formulated concealers designed to come to your rescue – whether it's a period zit or a large port-wine stain. Similarly, dark skins tend to heal very aggressively, leaving a deep-coloured scar – whether from acne or a bad cut – and a good camouflage base is often far more effective than so-called 'fader creams'.

Finding a product to suit you can be very much a matter of trial and error. Choose a concealer in the same way we suggest you choose a foundation, but go a shade lighter than your normal skin tone.

Generally you'll find concealers in either *tubes*, *wands*, *sticks* or *pots*. TUBES and WANDS contain liquid concealer which spreads very easily. This type is good for covering dark shadows under and around the eyes, broken veins, and the odd spot (we've used a wand in picture 5, page 28).

STICKS – a solid form of concealer, useful for the same sort of problems. Apply with a brush, not directly from the stick.

POTS usually contain the concealer suitable for heavy-duty camouflage jobs: scars, large birthmarks, port-wine stains and keloids. These require specialist concealers which aren't as widely available as the other types of camouflage . . . that's why we've got a comprehensive list of stockists in the 'Where to find it' section (page 85).

Camouflage make-up was originally developed during the First and Second World Wars for soldiers who had suffered terrible burns and scars.

applying

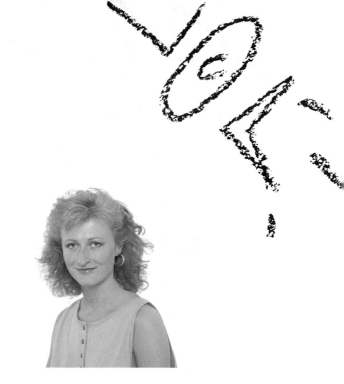

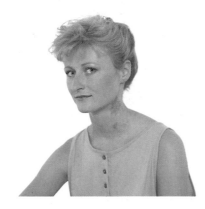

Tie your hair back and use a well-lit mirror, just as you would for an ordinary make-up. Cleanse, tone and moisturise your skin – making absolutely sure that the moisturiser has 'disappeared' into your skin completely. If any seems to remain on the surface, blot it with a tissue – otherwise you could find your make-up slip-sliding away! Camouflage creams are thicker and 'tackier' than ordinary foundations, so dab on a little at a time using your fingertips or a brush.

Work from the centre outwards until the blemish is covered, then 'set' with a translucent loose powder. Give yourself plenty of time, although it's a bit trickier to apply than normal base, it won't take you too long to get the hang of it. And the good news is that most camouflage bases are weatherproof, so, if you have a blemish that you find embarrassing, swimming or playing sports need no longer be an ordeal.

sculpting ~ coming next

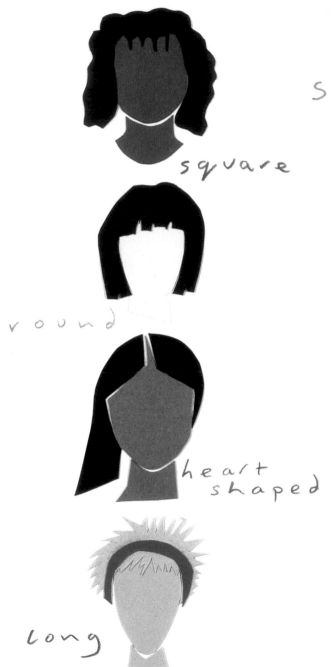

square

round

heart shaped

long

If you're happy with the shape of your face – fine. If not, blushers, shaders and highlighters can be used to create the *illusion* of a bone structure you never knew you had.

Think back to the questionnaire – what shape is your face? If the answer is 'not sure', stand in front of the mirror, hair pulled back and, with a soft pencil or an old lipstick, draw round your face shape as it appears in the mirror . . . Hey presto! There's the shape. Most faces come fairly close to one of four basic shapes: round, square, long, heart-shaped.

Could any of these possibly be you?!? In just a minute we'll tell you how to conjure up some pretty nifty illusions that should help to bring out the best in your face. In the meantime – the RAW MATERIALS:

BLUSHER – as the name suggests, it gives your cheeks a tinge of healthy-looking colour. You can also use it as a complete face-shaper if you want a very natural no-make-up look. Up until the sixties blusher was called 'rouge', which

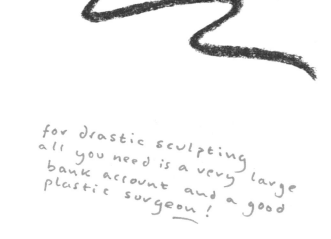

is just what it usually was – plain simple red. But nowadays blushers can be anything from the palest pink to the deepest burgundy. Your choice of colour will depend on your skin tone, your personality and your clothes.

SHADER – this is used to create shadows on your face and so it should be one or two tones darker than your natural skin tone.

HIGHLIGHTER – very light in colour, it can be shiny or matt and is used to emphasise, or create the illusion of, bone structure.

All three can be bought as creams, gels and compressed powder. Creams and gels should be applied after you've put on your foundation (if you use any), but *before* you put on your powder. Powder blusher should be applied on top of your face powder. The colour of these make-ups can look very dense in their containers, so always test them on your skin before buying . . . and never trust the colour shown on the outside of the package.

for drastic sculpting all you need is a very large bank account and a good plastic surgeon!

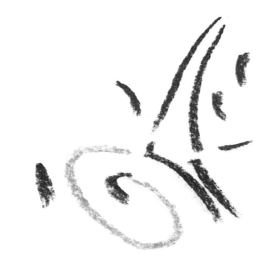

and now . . . applying

applying blusher

Once you've had a good look at your face, give it a good prod! It's only by feeling the contours that you'll be certain where to put your make-up. Feel the shape of your cheekbone area carefully. The blusher should go along the bone in a tear drop shape. A big rounded brush will make the application of powder blusher very easy. Brush the colour lightly, outwards along the bone. For a natural healthy look, fade the colour out before your hairline begins. If you bear in mind that a blusher is actually meant to imitate your natural blush, use *that* colour as a guideline when buying. Pale pinks and peach colours won't blend in happily with a dark or tanned skin tone, but will be perfect for paler skins. Similarly, brick or coppery reds will make a fair skin positively feverish – but will look great on dark skins.

By the way, if you're going to wear a brightly-coloured outfit, you may find you need more blusher than usual. If you're very dark skinned or rosy cheeked you probably won't want blusher at all.

Some suggestions for choosing colours:

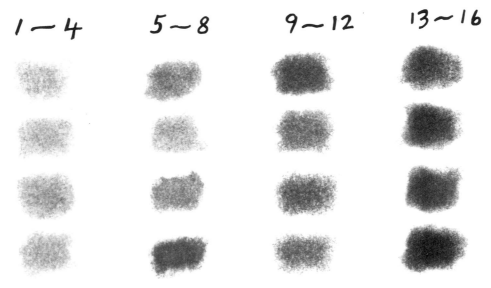

1 — 4   5 ~ 8   9 ~ 12   13 ~ 16

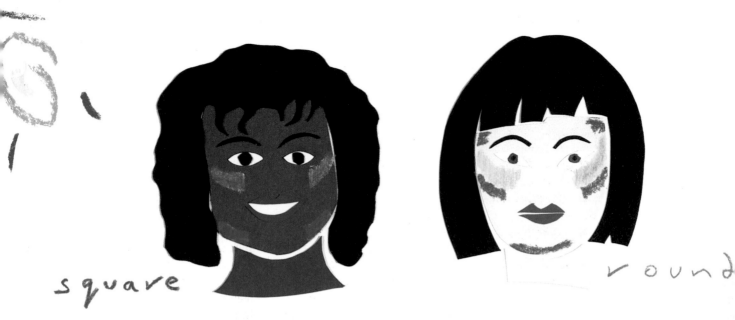

square

round

Before we show you some devilishly clever tricks you can perform, we'll now give you . . . ways to use shaders and highlighting to bring out the best in your face: round-long-square-heart-shaped.

highlighter

shader

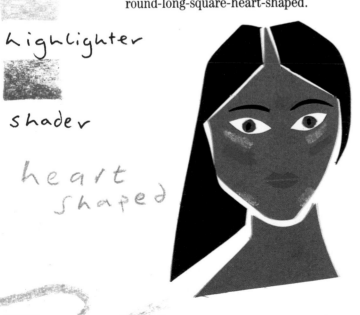

heart shaped

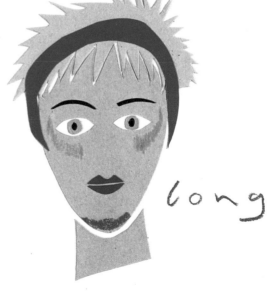

long

eyes right

eyes...
buying

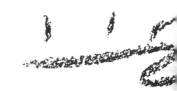

Own up – how long have you been wearing the same old colour on your eyelids? To quote that old proverb, 'the eyes are the windows of the soul', they are often the most animated part of your face and deserve your attention. But the endless conflicting advice and opinions on eye make-up, coupled with the vast number of products on the market, can be daunting, at the very least, and completely off-putting at worst. The trick is to tread the fine line between being brave and adventurous, without ending up broke.

Here's a checklist of the products you'll find on the shelves:

EYE SHADOWS – they can be sparkly or matt, and come in four forms: compressed powder, loose powder, cream and pencils.

Compressed powder is the most popular and the easiest to apply. It's quite useful to buy the sets of three – dark, medium and light in the colour of your choice. They can then be blended and 'graduated' with a brush for a contouring effect.

Loose powder is often sparkly, often sold in pots or wands and often ends up everywhere except on your eyelids! *But* if you're a sparkly type, then they really are the best. Different shades of loose powder can be successfully mixed before applying.

Creams come in tubes or pots and can be messy – they're apt to drift into the little creases in your eyes. But they are recommended for contact-lens wearers as they cause no irritation.

Soft, fat pencils are usually simply cream in a wooden pencil container, although there are some very powdery iridescent versions creeping onto the market. Pencils, as eye *shadows*, must be soft enough not to drag across your skin, but firm enough to be sharpened.

EYE LINER – comes in three forms – pencil, cake and liquid.

Pencils. The most popular colours for eye liner pencils are black, brown or grey, but they are now available in all kinds of zappy colours like purple, green and blue. Pencils should always be

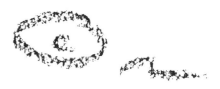

sharpened to give an even 'unblobby' line around your eyes, which can then be softened slightly with a brush. It's worth mentioning 'kohl' (Egyptian spelling) or 'Kajal' (Indian spelling) here. In this country it's usually sold in pencil form and can be used not only as an eye *liner*, but 'smudged' into an eye shadow and is also safe enough to use to line the inner rim of your eyelid. Black kohl pencil used in this way will emphasise the whites of your eyes, whilst a blue one will camouflage tired red rims.

Cake liner must be bought together with a fine applicator brush. It's very good for a definite line.

Liquid liners come in small bottles with their own little brushes (like nail varnish) and give a harder-edged look. Best for people with a steady hand.

MASCARA – you can buy mascara in almost any combination of 'natural-looking', 'lash-building' and/or water-proof. Bear in mind that people with contact lenses or those with sensitive eyes should steer clear of the lash-build-ing variety, as it contains small fibres which irritate the eyes. All types of mas-cara can be bought in wands, and natural-looking mascara can also be bought in cake form. It's applied, slightly dampened, with a small stiff brush, usually sold with the cake. Like eye liners – black, brown and also navy tend to be the most popular colours – but there is an increasing number of incredibly whacky shades around.

EYE-BROW PENCILS – these are the hardest pencils of all. They should be kept sharp and should match the natural colour of your eyebrows.
A quick word about eye make-up 'kits'. Often so-called 'complete' eye make-up sets are put together for you by the cos-metics manufacturer. They can appear to contain everything you need at a much more reasonable price. *If* you can honestly say that there's nothing in the kit that you *don't* need or like, then great. But be sure you're not falling prey to a devious plot to off-load some naff colours or end-of-the-range stock.

more eyes next ...

colours eyes... applying

If you're struggling with which colours to choose for your eyes, start off by experimenting with basic earthy tones, which are in fact much more like shader colours. These will blend in with, and suit, any eye colour, whether brown, grey, green or blue.

The idea of blue eye shadow for blue eyes is oldfashioned, and unflattering and doesn't make your eyes look as blue as brown eye shadow does! The important factors when choosing eye shadow colours are your hair colour and skin tone. Natural earthy colours are the most successful for learning how to shape and emphasise your eyes. When you're feeling braver you can try using brighter colours to match your clothes and the mood you're in.

If you're wearing base and powder – fine; you're ready to put on your eye make-up. If not, it's best to give yourself some kind of foundation to work on, and a light covering of base and powder really is best. It may seem fussy, but it'll help to even the colour, prevent creasing, make application much easier and all your work will last a lot longer.

The way you apply your make-up will depend entirely on the shape of your eyes – so it will be slightly different for everyone. But, generally speaking, your lid and browbone should be emphasised with a light colour and the socket should be deepened and shaded with a darker colour. To apply eye liner properly, draw it as closely as you can to your lashes; fade away where the lashes end for a natural look. For extra emphasis, you can put a softer line of darker eye shadow just under your bottom lashes, as close to your eye as possible.

As we've said, choosing colours is largely a matter of personal taste. But here are a few suggestions encompassing most skin tones.

1 ~ 4

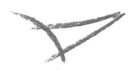

When putting on mascara, hold a small hand-mirror just below your eyes as you apply it to the top lashes – pushing the colour from the roots to the tips. Hold the mirror higher to see your bottom lashes and do the same. Comb away those little blobs with an eyelash comb, and use a cotton bud to clean up any accidents.

This is a very general guide to successfully applying eye make-up, but here are some suggestions for different-shaped eyes...

SMALL EYES – keep it light and subtle. Don't use dark kohl pencils inside your eyes and be careful with the mascara, as too much will only make your lashes look too heavy, closing up your eyes.

Contour your eyes by using a medium shade at the inner corner of your eyelid, a light colour in the centre and a darker one on the outer edge – never let the darkest of your three colours go in any further than the centre of your eyelid.

5 ~ 8   9 ~ 12   13 ~ 16

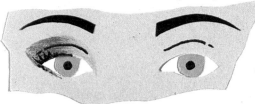

small

PROMINENT EYES – avoid pale or sparkly eye shadow on your lids – stick to darker matt shades. Use a medium tone in the sockets, not a darker one.

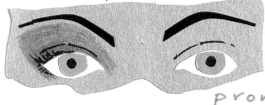

prominent

39

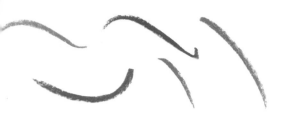

CLOSE-SET EYES – to create the illusion of more space between your eyes, always use very light shades on the inner corners of your lids – graduating to the darkest colour on the outer edge. Darken the outer corners of your eyes with a smudgy pencil (try kohl) in a V-shape around the corners.

DOWN-TURNED EYES – this type of eye shape can look a bit sad if you accentuate the wrong bits. So, try to blend your colours from mid to medium to darker tones in an upwards horizontal slant towards the outer edge.

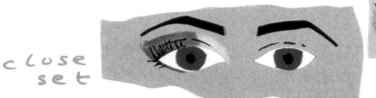

close set

down turn

WIDE APART EYES – the principle is the same as for close-set eyes, but in reverse – using a darker colour on the inner corners, blending to a lighter shade on the outer edge.

ORIENTAL-SHAPED – oriental-shaped eyes don't necessarily have a socket line. Although one can be shaded-in to give a 'western' look, it's equally valid to divide the eye vertically using lighter shades on the inner corners, graduating to darker shades at the edges. Use an eye liner to emphasise the almond shape.

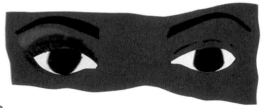

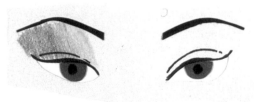

wide apart

oriental

eyebrows

Eyebrows define the shape of your eyes, complementing your make-up – so don't forget about them. Having made-up your eyes, brush away any stray foundation or eye shadow in the direction your eyebrows naturally grow. If your eyebrows tend to grow downwards, you can get a more flattering shape by brushing a little hair gel through them with an eyebrow brush or an old toothbrush in an upwards direction. Don't overdo the upwards bit, though, because you may end up looking permanently shocked!

To define your brows, or fill in any bald patches, you can use a hint of mascara or a sharp eyebrow pencil. Remember to use tiny light strokes going in the same direction, rather than a solid line. Keep checking that you are applying the same amount of eyebrow pencil to each eye.

There is no such thing as a perfectly-shaped eyebrow, as fashions and styles change continually, but if you come across any Denis Healey-type stragglers you can always pluck them away. For advice on plucking your eyebrows see page 70.

More than any other part of your face, your eyes reflect your general state of mind and body. Protect them well. For example, always wear goggles if you're using machinery, drilling or working with any toxic fluid which gives off fumes (paint, varnish, etc). Don't strain your eyes in too little light when reading or doing close work. Similarly, wear dark glasses in bright sunlight or bright reflected light. Don't watch the telly in the dark – always have another light on in the room, as the glare is too strong. Keep the brightness down on computer screens as well.

Never ignore headaches which could be caused by eye strain – see your doctor or an optician immediately.

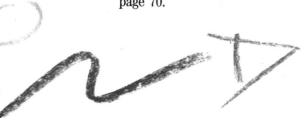

specs

Gone are the days of embarrassment specs-wise. They're now a fashion accessory in their own right. If you still loathe the very thought of them, most people can wear contact lenses – though the soft 24-hour variety are not recommended by many doctors.

As far as eye make-up and specs are concerned, remember that the glasses worn by long-sighted people make your eyes look bigger, which is very flattering, but keep your make-up tidy as every little blob will be magnified. If you're short-sighted your specs may make your eyes look smaller, so follow the advice for making up small eyes.

Choose your frames to suit your skin tone and the shape of your face. Here's a rough guide:

Pale-skinned people should go for warm colours – browns and reds.

Darker-skinned people should try blues, greys and paler frames.

Sallow and olive-skinned people should avoid gold and yellow frames.

If you've got a round face, wear square glasses with a strong horizontal line.

Square-shaped faces look best with curved Fifties-style glasses – wider than the face. Avoid obvious square and rectangular shapes.

Long faces can wear specs as wide as you like with strong square or rectangular frames.

If your face is heart-shaped, you can wear almost any frames apart from long deep ones.

When it comes to sunglasses, in order to be effective they should filter 85% of the light. How do you tell? Look in the mirror (with your sunspecs on, of course!) – if you can still see your eyes, they're not strong enough.

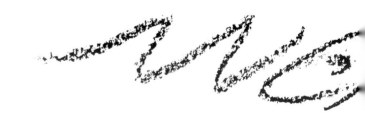

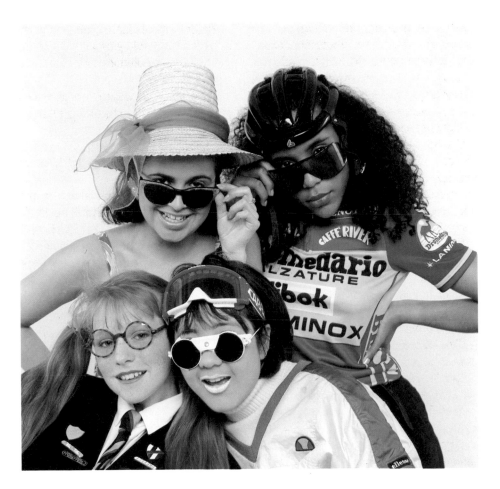

lips to follow

buying
lipstick

applying

Lip colours come in pots, sticks, wands, palettes and pencils. They are manufactured in an astounding variety of colours and finishes – including pearly, matt and glossy. Lip pencils are normally used for outlining the shape of your mouth, but can be used for filling in as well, if they're the softer, fatter type.

Lipstick is a cosmetic with which you can go wild, experimenting with all sorts of colours – matching or clashing with your clothes to create any number of effects. First, some money-saving tips:

Buy a cheap paint palette or a clear plastic bobbin-holder box in which you can collect, mix and match different brands and colours together.

Don't be fooled into paying high prices for fancy packaging – you don't wear the package on your face, after all!

Always have a colourless lip gloss or vaseline in your make-up bag. By adding it in varying amounts to any matt lipstick, you can create depths of colour to suit your needs – whether it's a hint of colour for work or school, or a vibrant, glossy look for parties.

1 Outline the natural shape of your lips with a sharpened lip pencil. It should be the same colour as your lipstick or your natural lip colour.

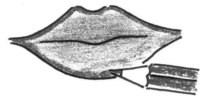

2 Fill in with lip colour using a square-ended brush. Stretch your lips into a smile, so you fill in all the little cracks to get an even colour. Blend in the edges completely so there's no obvious line.

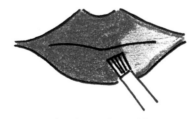

For long-lasting colour, blot your lips by pressing a tissue between them, powder lightly and apply a second coat of lipstick.

1 ~ 4

5 ~ 8

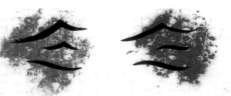
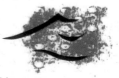

Dark-skinned girls may have a darker top lip than bottom lip. This can be evened out by applying a dark lipstick or a base to your bottom lip, matching the tone of your top lip. You can then put a coloured lipstick over the whole lot.

fuller lips

How to make your lips look fuller: Apply base and powder over your lips. Use a lip liner *just* on the outside of your natural line, and then fill in. Go for glossy and frosted lipsticks, as darker, more matt finishes will make your lips look thinner – giving a hard, mean look.

smaller lips

How to make your lips look smaller: just the same, but use the lip liner just inside your natural line and fill in with colour. Avoid pearly and glossy lipsticks and bright colours, which will make lips look fuller.

If you have a much fuller top lip than bottom, or vice versa, fill out the thinner lip as above.

By the way, when you've painted on those perfect lips – the effect could be ruined when you smile . . . if you don't take care of your teeth. Regular dental check-ups (twice a year) are a must. Even the ritziest red lipstick won't hide bad teeth.

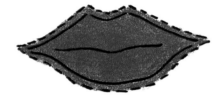

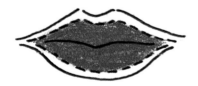

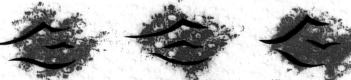

hands

'You need hands . . . ' and it doesn't take long to keep them in good condition. Washing your hands causes dryness; always use a hand cream afterwards. If your hands are always in the sink or doing messy jobs, use a barrier cream or petroleum jelly. And remember detergents are bad for your hands so wear rubber gloves.

Nothing can ruin a glamorous look like gungy bits under the nails, worse still, no nails at all (stop biting them this instant!) and chipped nail polish. If you suffer from weak nails, nail nourishers and hardeners can help. It could also be due to a diet deficiency, so step up your calcium intake. If you bite your nails, you could buy an evil-tasting anti-nail-biting lotion or, better still, enrol for some relaxing yoga classes!

To keep your nails in good shape soak the fingertips in a bowl of warm, soapy water to loosen any dirt under the tips and to soften the cuticles. Dry the nails and clean the underside with an orange stick. Using the blunt end of the orange stick, gently push back the cuticles.

Trim very long nails with clippers or nail scissors then file into shape – in one direction only – using an emery board, not a metal file. Don't file too deeply at the corners, aim for straight sides and a slightly rounded top. Buff nails for a natural shine, in one direction again.

If you want to apply new varnish, always start with clean hands and nails. Remove any old bits of varnish with nail polish remover. Acetone is the main ingredient of removers, but don't be tempted to use it neat as it is too harsh and drying on its own. Use a cotton bud for the awkward bits of varnish left in the corners. On the market there are base coats which should be used first as a protective undercoat. Apply thinly and allow to dry thoroughly. Apply the nail colour next. One stroke in the centre of the nail then one along each side to coat the nail completely. Don't backtrack over any missing bits. Instead apply a second coat when the first is completely dry. There are sprays and 'dryers' available which do this quickly, if you are in a hurry.

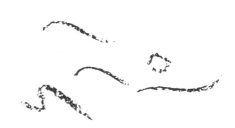

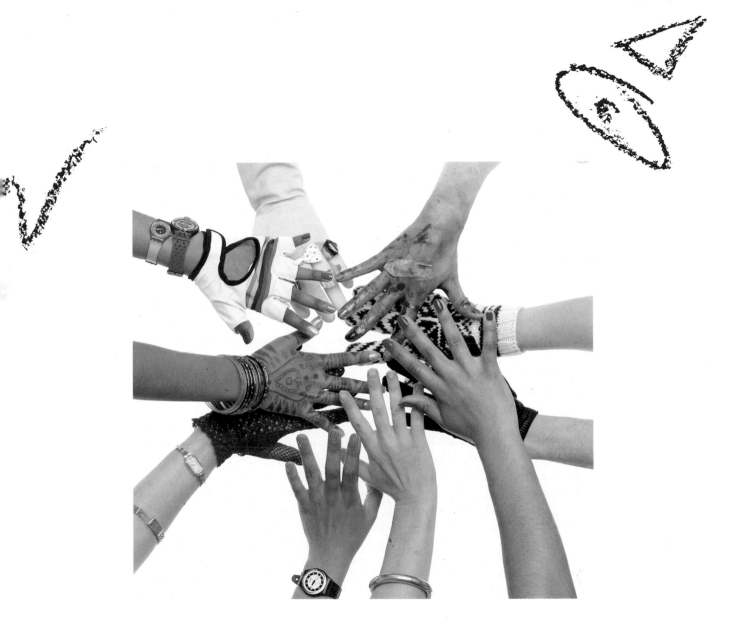

looking good.

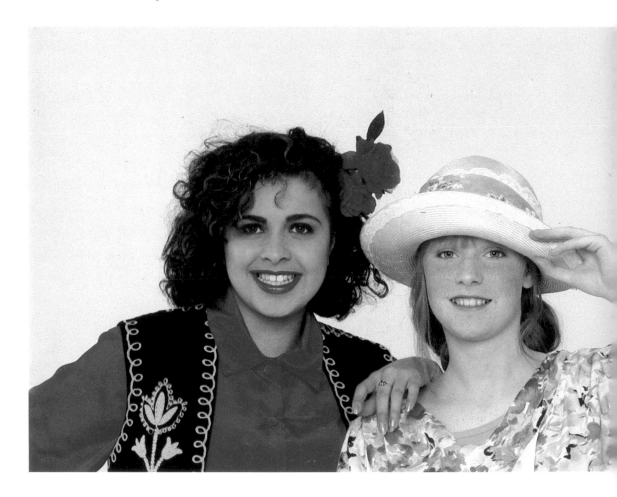

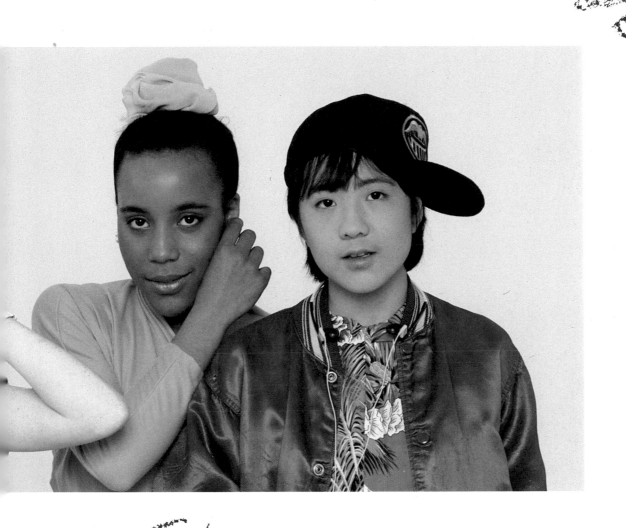

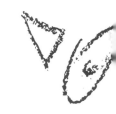

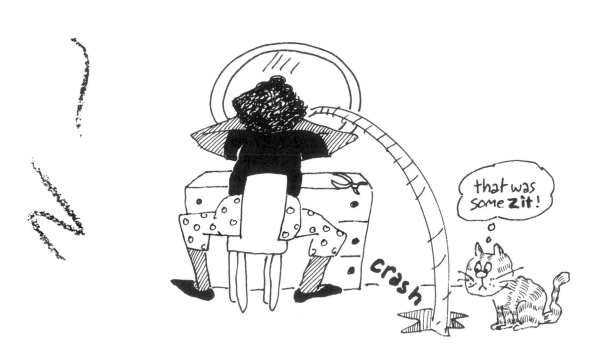

general maintenance

- tool maintenance
- skin maintenance
- body maintenance
  - treats
  - problems

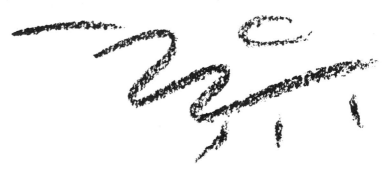

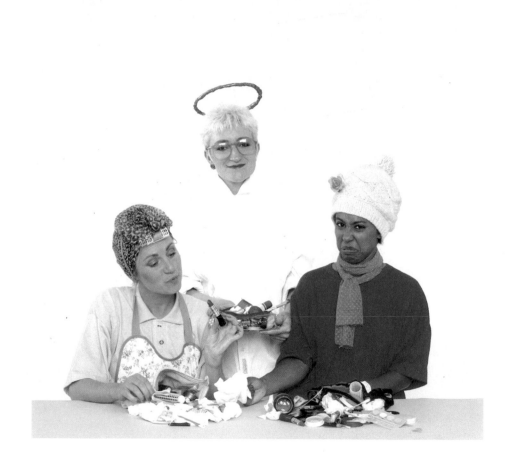

the art of tool maintenance

Yuk! Confess – would *you* be ready and willing to show your make-up bag to the world? Is *your* make-up bag a disgusting, sticky mess? Shame on you! Or is it a shining example of which any professional make-up artist would be proud? How can you hope to create a sparkling new 'you' if your brushes are still covered in last week's gunk?

Always clean sponges, puffs and brushes in a mild solution of detergent, or soap, and warm water. Rinse very thoroughly. Press your brushes gently back into shape with your fingers and stand them upright in a jar (bristles uppermost of course!) to dry. Good quality brushes are invaluable and deserve your respect. If your make-up mirror is covered in sticky fingermarks, clean it with a drop of meths on a tissue.

As a rule, people carry around far too much make-up and this only makes the yukky make-up bag factor worse. Tops, lids and caps have a habit of working loose – jumbling everything together beautifully. Ring any bells? Keep most of your make-up at home in a tin or box (a biscuit tin or small fishing tackle box is ideal), next to your make-up mirror. This is much more practical than a big lumpy bag. Find a jar or a pot suitable for standing your brushes in.

Carry around the minimum of make-up – just enough for quick retouching jobs. Choose a practical, washable make-up bag and keep it clean. Clear see-through pencil cases are cheaper and easier to use than padded fabric.

Finally, NEVER swap tools or eye and lip make-up. It's unhygienic and could pass on infection.

the back of your hand is a great palette for mixing colours.

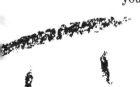

skin maintenance

wrinkles will appear eventually for the same reason that a pavement will get cracks ~ time and wear ~

humid and island climates bring out the best in skin ~ british, scandinavian, fijian and polynesian races are renowned for healthy youthful skin ~

Just as 'what goes up must come down', so 'what goes on must come off'! This not only applies to make-up...your poor old face is bombarded with dirt and pollution, especially if you live in a big town or city. Whether or not you use make-up, it's very important to keep your skin clean and healthy with a good cleansing routine.

What is skin? It actually consists of two layers: the *dermis*, where cells are created and pushed up to the surface, and the *epidermis*, which provides an impenetrable layer against germs and bacteria – unless it's cracked or cut. It takes 21–28 days for new cells to work upwards and shed themselves on the sur-face of the epidermis. This is why it often takes a few weeks for a change of diet or skin-care routine to show any visible difference.

Your skin also contains *sebaceous glands*, which produce natural body oil, and two different kinds of sweat glands which help to wash away excess oil and dust. The mixture of natural oil and sweat forms a protective 'acid mantle', which maintains the correct acid/alkali balance in your skin and protects against germs and other nasties. Be wary of products, particularly cleansers, that claim to balance out the so-called 'PH factor' of your skin – almost ALL products are automatically neutralized by your skin itself within an hour of use. However, this doesn't apply to soap, which needs to be thoroughly rinsed off.

Your choice of cleanser depends on your skin type, and this is determined by the amount of oil your sebaceous glands produce:

NORMAL SKIN is smooth with no enlarged pores.

DRY SKIN is flaky and may become red or sore in cold weather.

OILY SKIN is coarser in texture, with enlarged pores around the nose and chin. It often looks shiny and is more prone to spots.

COMBINATION SKIN is what most adults have, with dry skin on the cheeks and an oily panel down the forehead, nose and chin.

To determine your skin type, try the 'sticky-tape' test: smooth a piece of sticky-tape across your cheeks and nose, and then peel it off. If it doesn't stick very easily, then your skin is oily. If bits of skin flake off with it, then your skin is dry. If it's oily in the middle and flaky on the cheeks, then it's combination! Simple, eh?!

aloe vera ~ has many uses including healing burns ~ it is a gel extracted from a lily type flower.

coming clean next

cleansers

These come in a bewildering variety of forms, and with a staggering list of claims. The *only* guideline is to choose one which feels good on your skin. Some people swear by good old soap and water, while others find it leaves their skin with a very 'tight' feeling. However, the gentle rubbing motion with soap, water and a soft flannel can have a mildly exfoliating effect. This can be of particular benefit to people with dark skins, which shed their cells at a faster rate. However, soap and water by themselves are not sufficient to remove make-up, so use a cream cleanser beforehand, and a toner afterwards to remove any traces of soap. If you have a dry or sensitive skin, steer well clear of normal soaps – especially perfumed ones.

Cleansing lotions and creams are the only efficient way of removing make-up. As they are a mixture of oil and water, they literally 'float' make-up and grime off your face. For the best results, massage the lotion or cream well into the face with your fingertips, and remove with dampened tissue or cotton wool.

Make all the movements on your face gentle and never drag your skin, but use a circular motion in an upward and outward direction.

If you have a very dry skin, look for a moisturising cleanser as it will leave behind a thin film of moisturiser, like almond oil, for example.

Cleansers for oily skins contain ingredients like lemon juice and cucumber which help to keep those perky sebaceous glands in check!

Eyes and lips need special attention. The skin around your eyes is very delicate, so go easy. Remove your eye make-up first, using a special cleanser. The products on the market to remove eye make-up are usually very oily . . . baby oil is just as good, and completely safe. Apply it with a damp piece of cotton wool, stroking across the top of your eye, and then back inwards towards the inner corner. Don't drag the skin outwards or you'll end up with bags before your time! Also, leaving your mascara on overnight encourages tiny wrinkles to form – so take it off!!

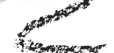

moisturisers

Go easy with moisturisers on your eyes, because too rich a mixture can cause puffiness. If you wear contact lenses, make sure you take them out before you take off your make-up – or they'll end up covered in gunk.

You can use your usual cleanser on lips, but don't use a face-pack or 'scrub' (more on those later!) near them.

toners

A good toner will finish off your cleansing routine by shifting any leftover bits of make-up and cleansing lotion, and closing up the pores of your skin. Apply with cotton wool, lightly dabbing it over your face – avoid your eyes. Toners are sometimes called 'astringents' or 'fresheners'. Astringents normally contain alcohol, which dries the skin, so they're ideal for oily skin, but dry and sensitive skins should always use alcohol-free products. Combination skins should *try* and use a mixture of toners: astringent on the oily bits and alcohol-free on the dry patches.

A moisturiser should protect a clean face and help to keep it supple. It forms a barrier, easing the effects of cold, wind and central heating, as well as providing a protective base for make-up. ALL skin types need moisturiser, but there are nearly as many around as there are skins! Again, it's a case of finding the one that suits you and sticking with it. Whilst being wary of extravagant claims, no moisturiser can work miracles, it's worth knowing that creams containing Vitamin A can help acne, and those containing Vitamin E or Arnica can help scars to heal and improve your skin's ability to absorb moisture.

Use a moisturiser first thing in the morning and last thing at night, always after cleansing and toning, massaging it in gently from the centre of your face outwards. If you have a particularly dry skin you could try using a richer 'night cream' at bedtime . . . but don't put it on your eyes. However oily a skin you may have, don't be tempted to skip using a very light moisturiser . . . think of it as protection.

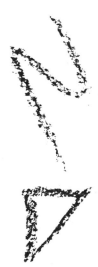

sun . . . sun . . . sun

sun creams and sun screens   body maintenance

Your long-suffering skin not only has to withstand overheated rooms, cold winds, pollution and acid rain, but periodically it's subjected to being fried in the scorching rays of the sun. Unfortunately, the experts have only one attitude towards sunbathing: DON'T DO IT! But, in real life, who can resist scampering out into the sunshine once in a while? On the good side, your skin needs to absorb Vitamin D from the sun.

Fair skin burns very easily and should always be protected from the sun with a barrier cream. Follow the instructions carefully, only ever using creams, lotions or oils which carry detailed information and instructions with the product. Even darker skins need some protection, so use a light barrier cream. Whatever your skin type, stay out of the mid- day sun!

Ultra-violet nasties can also be reflected off water and snow. Studies in the US show that snow reflects 87% of the sun's rays, as opposed to 17% from sand – so beware! Protect yourself with a high-protection barrier cream if you're thinking of going skiing or sailing.

Before moving on to 'treats' and goodies for your face, a few handy hints on looking after your whole body! It's no good sticking on your slap over a face mistreated by too many sticky buns, late nights and cigarettes. Exercise, good diet plus lots of relaxation and rest are as important as a good skin-care routine.

The simplest exercise can be an anti-dote to feeling wound-up and tense; a brisk walk or jog to work, school or the shops can work wonders. Swimming and cycling also provide great all-round exercise. Whenever possible, try to find time to relax: a warm bath before bed, putting your feet up with a cup of tea and a good book or even just shutting your eyes and breathing deeply for a few minutes – all of these can be very therapeutic.

As for diet, most of us eat far too much fat, sugar and salt – but not enough fibre-rich foods, fresh fruit and vegetables. The body needs those essential vitamins and minerals to help fight off zits and bags. Vitamin C intake is especially important as our bodies are unable to store it. By the way, if you're on the Pill you can only absorb Vitamin C in its natural form, e.g. all citrus fruits, strawberries, peppers, cauliflower, cabbage and potatoes cooked in their jackets. The three other essential skin vitamins are: Vitamin A, found in carrots, watercress and parsley; Vitamin E, found in nuts, beans and wheatgerm; and Vitamin D, absorbed through the skin from sunshine and found in butter, fish, eggs and milk. Important minerals include calcium and zinc, which can be taken in tablet form.

If you've got problem skin, steer clear of tea and coffee and try herb teas instead. Wholemeal flour products are rich in B vitamins which help any dry skin conditions.

As for those fats . . . well, what can we say? Whether or not they actually cause spots is open to debate – but they certainly add to the double chins. Try using skimmed milk and low-fat spreads. Grill or bake your food rather than frying it.

Finally, sugar: the average British person eats A POUND OF SUGAR A DAY!!! Cut down on sugar in tea and coffee, drink unsweetened fruit juice and try to ration sticky buns and chocolate bars. Sugar is addictive – so train those tastebuds to do without!

Remember, though, not all 'convenience foods' are bad for you. Tinned fish, tomatoes and beans are all very healthy, as are frozen fish and peas (in fact frozen peas often contain more vitamins than fresh ones). Dried beans and cereals are also full of farty fibre . . .

never be tempted to skip breakfast it's the most important fuel of the day

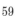

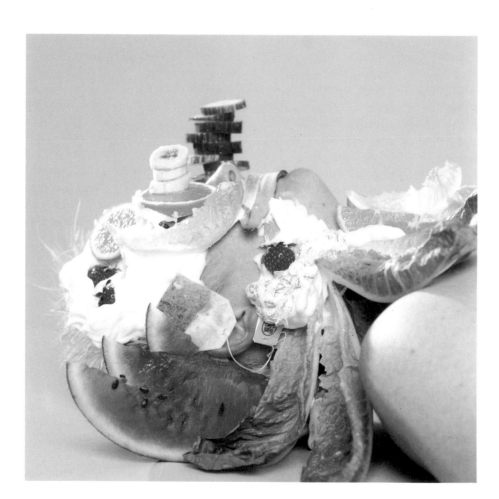

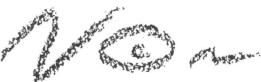

treats

Your skin deserves treats. Pollution, central heating, air conditioning, processed food and preservatives are all part of everyday modern living and are all bad for your complexion. The right diet, mineral water and regular exercise are 'inner' cleansers that will help to redress the balance. But there is no harm in taking the time to pamper yourself with treats that can be applied to the 'outside' as well! There are all sorts of treatments for your skin that will cleanse, moisturise, tone and even improve minor ailments – at the same time as relaxing you and improving your general sense of well-being.

Many of these treatments have been used by women for centuries, the recipes varying according to climate, demands and what kind of 'materials' were available. As these materials were usually vegetables, fruit, flowers and herbs, with the aid of refrigeration we can all now swap and benefit from each other's ideas. These types of treats tend to be very much 'Do It Yourself' jobs – cheap, fun to try out and very satisfying.

There are treats to be had for serious money, if you have the cash and the inclination. If you don't feel like splashing out on yourself, you could always get someone else to spend *for* you as a birthday present, for example.

Before moving on to the really expensive stuff, a quick word about 'semi-D.I.Y.' treatments. These are ready-made preparations you can buy from stores and chemists and they include: face packs, face gels and exfoliating 'scrubs'. The latter aren't as painful as they sound! A 'scrub' will actually remove the dead cells from the surface of your skin and, with regular use, will restore a healthy glow.

Most manufactured face packs and gels contain ingredients which draw out the toxins and excess oils, tightening the skin and closing the pores. This leaves your face feeling smoother and refreshed. Many cosmetics ranges also manufacture their own skin-care products. As well as cleansers, moisturisers and toners they also produce lotions and potions claiming to per-

more treats to come

form every trick imaginable, from eradicating early wrinkles to – wait for it – bleaching dark skin paler!!! That's an extreme example, but do watch out for the 'you-didn't-know-you-had-a-problem-until-we-told-you' syndrome.

Now for the treats that are completely devoid of any D.I.Y. – you simply lie back, think of 'wherever' and try *not* to think of how much it's costing! We are, of course, talking about the wonderful world of BEAUTY SALONS . . . !

Now, beauty salons *can* seem like frightening and mysterious places run by regiments of crisply-dressed, ever-smiling, perfectly manicured 'therapists', who offer strange and tortuous-sounding treatments like 'geloide prescription facials', 'cathiodermie neck treatment' and mechanical massage for cellulite. *But*, if you are feeling extravagant and in need of pampering, there is much pleasure to be had and much infc to be gleaned from just one visit. For a start, the therapists train long and hard – and they know their stuff. Normally they're only too willing to impart all sorts of handy hints, whilst completing your treatment to perfection. Most beauty salons will offer treatments for your face and separate treatments for your body like massage, steam baths, back scrubs, waxing, pedicures and manicures, sunbeds and sometimes aromatherapy and reflexology.

Facial treatments usually include:

Removing unwanted facial hair by waxing, electrolysis or plucking (the latter only for eyebrow shaping).

Eyebrow and eyelash tinting (normally lasts for about six weeks).

Advice and ideas on your personal make-up.

Full facial, involving deep cleansing, steaming, blackhead and spot clearance, a face pack and lots of lovely massage. Bliss!

It's difficult to quote prices here, but at the time of writing a personal make-up instruction session varied from £40.00 to £12.95. These are London prices and this would be a one-off session, unlike a facial, which ranged from £25.00 to £11.75. Look for bargains . . . all salons have little handouts quoting their treatments and price lists. So take one away with you and study it before committing yourself. Beauty salons are often situated in or near to hairdressing salons – run as a separate part of the same business. This is often the case in department stores and high-street salons. Sometimes they are run as shops in their own right and occasionally they can be found in health clubs. Don't feel intimidated about going in – it doesn't cost anything to ask a few questions.

treats you can make

Now, at last, the real grassroots stuff! The completely 'Do It Yourself' methods that have been used by our foremothers for centuries.

Good diet and good looks go hand in hand, so it makes sense that we should put good natural products on our bodies as well as inside them. Women around the world have always used natural herbs, fruit and vegetables to soothe and soften the skin. In the twentieth century we have proved scientifically that these products contain essential vitamins, minerals, proteins and oils to invigorate your system inside and out!

In fact, many expensive and sophisti-cated skin treatments contain natural products and it's often much cheaper and just as good to raid the fridge and concoct your own!

Coming up now are some tried and trusted skin treats and a few simple recipes. As always, feel free to experi-ment with your own combinations to find out what best suits you!

old favourites

HONEY – one of the earliest known skin treatments used as a skin softener. Use it on its own as a mask or try mixing: 1 tablespoon of clear honey with 1 table-spoon of ground almonds as a face scrub (suitable for all skin types). Also, 1 tea-spoon in the bath will rejuvenate and soothe.

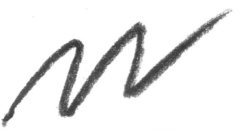

YOGHURT – a great all-rounder! The Greeks used it for sunburn. It's also great as a soothing face mask. For dry skin a good face mask is a mixture of yoghurt, 1 tablespoon of oatmeal and a squeeze of lemon. Leave it on for ten minutes and rinse off with cold water.

CUCUMBER – again has been used for centuries to soothe and cool. While you're relaxing with a face pack, put a few slices on your eyelids to refresh your eyes. Cucumber lotion (blend cucumber and a little water together in a blender and strain) is excellent for sore skin or sunburn.

STRAWBERRIES – rich in Vitamin C and also excellent for sunburn. Crushed and put on the face they make an excellent mask for oily skin.

AVOCADO – rich in Vitamins A and B and good for all skin types. After you've eaten one, rub the inside of the skin over your face, leave for a few minutes and rinse off with cool water.

ROSEWATER – you can buy this cheaply in big bottles from most chemists and healthfood shops. It's been used for over 2000 years as a skin freshener and toner. For a more astringent effect (needed with oily skin), try mixing: 75 ml rose water with 25 ml witch hazel (also from chemists).

LEMON JUICE – again, great inside and out! A natural antiseptic and astringent (for oily skin). The juice of a lemon in a cup of hot water gets the system going in the morning. On your face it has excellent bleaching properties and can be used to bleach facial hairs.

OILS – wheatgerm oil and Vitamin E oil, again both available from healthfood shops and chemists, are rich in Vitamin E – the vitamin which helps heal skin, and which is particularly good for scars. Use as a face massage oil. Also for clean smooth hands, gently rub a little olive oil and granulated sugar over your hands for a few minutes and then wash off.

OATMEAL – good for face scrubs, just add it to your own cream cleanser.

HERBS – an infusion of camomile or sage makes an excellent skin freshener. To make an infusion add one tablespoon of the herb to a cup of hot water – leave to stand and cool then strain. This liquid can be kept for several days in the fridge. Add herbs to your bath water too (tie some up in a little muslin or cotton bag): camomile to soothe and relax; pepper-mint, rosemary or thyme to invigorate.

WATER – yes, there's nothing quite like good old tap water! Cold water splashed over the face makes a brilliant toner to close those pores. Try filling a plant spray with mineral water and keeping it in the fridge. Spray your face to freshen it and also to set your make-up (much cheaper than expensive aerosols!).

FULLER'S EARTH – (from chemist) mixed with egg white and water makes a great face pack for all skin types. Leave for a few minutes and rinse off.

a do it yourself facial

A facial will relax you whilst cleansing, nourishing and toning your skin. Give yourself plenty of time and follow these instructions:

Tie back your hair, or if it's very short, keep it back with a stretch bandage.

Steam your face using a herbal infusion – pour the heated infusion into a basin and lean over it with your head under a towel, keeping your face about 12″ away from the basin.

Blot away the excess moisture from your face and gently put on your face mask. Use your fingertips, taking care not to 'drag' your skin. Avoid the area around your eyes and mouth.

Cover your eyes either with gauze or cotton wool pads soaked in a cold herbal infusion, or with thin slices of cucumber. Now be very quiet and still. Don't let anyone disturb you, just lie there and relax. Try not to speak or move your face as the mask will crack and won't be so effective. Leave for about 10 minutes. Wash off your face mask using cotton wool pads and luke-warm water. Put on a very thin layer of light moisturiser.

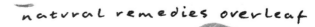
natural remedies overleaf

acne

Acne is normally associated with oily skin and is suffered by people of all ages – though it seems to affect all teenagers to some degree. This is due to the fact that hormone levels rise during adolescence and the sebaceous (oil-producing) glands become more active. In turn, there is an excess production of the top layer of skin cells which, along with oil, dust and dirt can block the ducts of these glands. Thereby appears a spot! The waxy plug blocking the skin pore forms a blackhead when it's exposed to the air . . . if it becomes infected – thereby appears another spot!! A blocked pore that is *not* exposed to the air forms a whitehead . . . (still there??)

Of course, the multi-million-dollar question about spots is: '*To squeeze or not to squeeze?*' There are many arguments 'against' and not so many 'for'. But let's face it, if you've got an interview, a wedding, a party or a hot date, you're sure as hell going to get a spot right where it shows – and you have to be a saint not to try and attack it there and then.

Firstly, consider the problems of squeezing. You can cause serious scarring – particularly if you have a dark skin. By pressing incorrectly you can make the spot *im*plode – with the walls of the infected duct bursting, causing further infection deep down in the skin. A 'cystic lesion' can follow, with permanent scarring, after the actual spot has healed.

So, what are the other solutions – apart from forking out money for a trained beauty therapist to squeeze your blackheads safely for you? Prevention? Well, there is no *absolute* proof that what you eat causes spots. However, a healthy balanced diet with the right mixture of fibre, vitamins, minerals, protein, fats *and* carbohydrates certainly isn't going to do your skin any harm. You may find that there's one particular food that triggers off spots: chocolate or ice cream maybe. Drink plenty of water – the bottled variety if you're not sure about the water in your area – this really does seem to help.

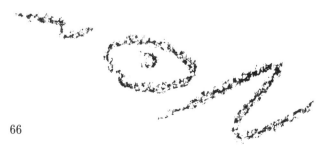

Exercise will cleanse your skin of excess waste products. Of course, try to keep your skin clean with a medicated soap, milk, lotion or cream – whichever you find suits you best. Don't wash more than twice a day... the sebaceous glands will be stimulated to produce more oil, the more you wash. Oil itself is not 'dirty' – it only becomes dirty and dangerous when you start picking and squeezing.

Sunshine or carefully regulated sessions under ultra-violet rays can both help to zap those zits and clear up acne. Other treatments include special preparations that you can buy from the chemist without prescription.

If your acne is severe there are more serious remedies which must be authorised by a doctor: antiseptic skin-peeling preparations; small, regular doses of antibiotics or even prolonged treatment with special drugs. Please don't forget about natural remedies, though. It might be worth investigating homeopathic treatments, which will cause none of the side-effects of antibiotics.

If you've suffered from chronic acne and you're now left with very angry-looking scars, you could consider a mild form of plastic surgery which removes the top layer of skin. Plastering heavy make-up on top of scars will only cause further blockage and more problems.

Has all this put you off sneaking in the odd squeeze? No? Well, then please be careful and thoroughly clean your skin first and cover your fingers and nails with cotton wool dampened with diluted antiseptic. Gently push your fingers together on either side of the zit. Only ever try to squeeze the spots and whiteheads that have come up *above* the surface – *never* touch the under-the-skin ones. And for heaven's sake, don't tell anyone we told you about this!!

eczema over the page

eczema

There are many different types of eczema, but these are the symptoms common to all sufferers: a sore rash, dry flaky skin and itchiness. Apart from that, eczema is an entirely individual condition, coming, going and sometimes disappearing altogether for no apparent reason. There is no instant cure and, as sufferers will know, many factors can act as a trigger: stress, anxiety, heredity, diet, allergy and sensitivity in general, cell formation as well as skin type. As each person's case is so different, advice and help must come from either a doctor or skin clinic.

Unlike many cases of acne, eczema is not associated with adolescence. So by the time someone suffering from eczema gets to the stage of wanting to try out make-up, they may already know which products suit them. However, if you're in any way unsure or confused, the National Eczema Society (address in the 'Where To Find It' section page 85) has a leaflet on skin care.

In the meantime, here are a few guidelines. There are some ingredients used in making cosmetics and toiletries which can irritate an already sensitive skin. For example, you'd be well advised to steer clear of sun-screens and hair-removing creams. It's largely a question of trial and error finding the specific cosmetics to suit you. Generally speaking, the following substances have been found to cause a bad reaction: natural perfume oil, orris root, indelible dyes, cornstarch, crude lanolin, certain resins, henna and herb compounds, cocoa butter and preservatives.

Hypo-allergenic cosmetics and skin-care products try to leave out most allergens and irritants, having been submitted to thorough laboratory and dermatological tests before reaching the shop counter. They also list the ingredients on the package so you know exactly what you'll be buying.

Before concluding on eczema, we'd like to recommend Christine Orton's book, *Eczema – A Complete Guide To All The Remedies – Alternative and Orthodox*.

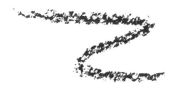

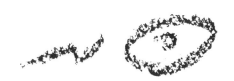

keloids

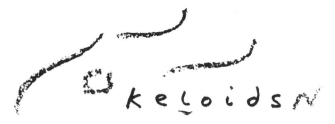

Black skin is very active when it comes to healing itself after an injury, a vaccination, a burn, an operation, or even ear-piercing. When the fibrous tissues that form a scar become excessive, a keloid is formed. Keloids are absolutely harmless – but they can look conspicuous. A doctor will be able to recommend the best way to get rid of them. This can involve either a series of injections to make the keloid smaller, cryosurgery (freezing the little devil off), radiotherapy or plastic surgery. A keloid cannot simply be cut off as it would leave another scar and therefore another keloid.

pigment increase and loss

These are problems mainly affecting dark skins. Pigment loss is usually noticed first on your hands and face, and is known as 'vitiligo'. Have a look at our 'Camouflage' section (page 30) for some truly magical cover-ups. It's best to avoid long exposure to the sun, as the pale patches will look even lighter when the rest of your skin becomes tanned.

Pigment *increase* is known medically as 'cholasma' and usually darkens the centre of your face, around your eyes and along your upper lip. Mostly, cholasma fades by itself, but it can take a while to disappear completely. If you've noticed any increase in your pigmentation and have any worries about it, see your doctor immediately. Whilst it heals itself, try out the concealers shown in the camouflage section and listed in the 'Where To Find It' section (page 85).

warts

These are small benign tumours of the skin. Often they can vanish without treatment, or they can be 'frozen' or removed chemically.

facial hair next

moles

Moles are raised, brown skin blemishes made up of a mass of cells with a high concentration of melanin (skin pigment). Some moles have little hairs growing out of them. These should not be plucked, in case of infection . . . try trimming them carefully with nail scissors instead. Normally, moles – sometimes referred to as 'beauty spots' – are harmless. Occasionally a mole becomes malignant, the signs being an increase in size, change in colour, bleeding or an ulcerous appearance. See your doctor straight away if you have any worries whatsoever or if you wish to have a mole surgically removed.

facial hair

Everyone has hair, however fine, growing on their face. Some people – depending on their hormone balance and colouring – have heavier, darker facial hair than others. There is *nothing* unnatural about this, unless it makes you feel unhappy or uncomfortable. Hairiness *can* be a temporary phase, whilst hormones are changing during adolescence (do you ever get the feeling life would be a lot easier without damn hormones?!?). In the meantime, there are all sorts of ways to get rid of unwanted facial hair.

If you feel your eyebrows are too heavy, with odd straggly ones and perhaps hairs growing on the bridge of your nose, pluck them carefully with broad-ended tweezers. Get the tweezers as close to the root of the hair as you can, pulling gently but firmly in the direction from which the hair is growing. If you're plucking your eyebrows for the first time, be wary of getting carried away . . . it's very easy, unless you stop and check in the mirror after plucking every couple of hairs, to end up completely browless with that shaved, Elizabeth the First look!!!

Try not to pluck your eyebrows directly before applying eye make-up as it can leave little red marks for a short time afterwards.

Here's a guide to good, naturally-shaped eyebrows . . .

Look in the mirror . . . take a pencil

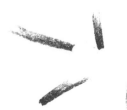

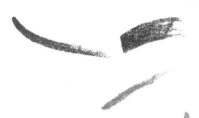

and hold it so it makes a line at the side of your nose and the inner corner of your eye. Follow that line upwards . . . where it crosses the line of your brow is exactly where the brow should start. Now hold the pencil at an angle from the side of your nose to the outer corner of your eye . . . the place where the pencil crosses your eyebrow is an ideal place for it to end.

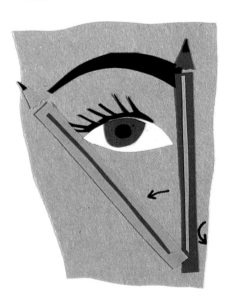

Lots of people's eyebrows aren't quite as long as this diagram would suggest. It doesn't matter – this is really a guide for when you're wearing make-up, so it won't look odd if you paint or draw in a few extra 'hairs' with a cake liner or a sharpened eyebrow pencil.

Don't ever be tempted to pluck or shave hairs on your chin, on the side of your face or on your upper lip. You can bleach these quickly and easily with preparations from the chemist, and the effect should last for several weeks.

The only permanent solution is electrolysis. Each hair is treated individually with a tiny needle and must be done by a qualified electrolysist. This treatment can be lengthy and expensive and is probably best postponed if you're still young because, as mentioned, it could be just temporary hairiness.

If you feel you have excessive facial hair, it could be a hormone imbalance and your doctor will be able to tell you if hormone therapy could help.

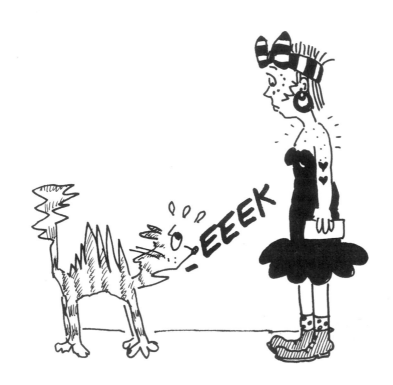

special effects

So far in this book we've concentrated on make-up that will enhance your own *natural* appearance, rather than turn you into a cloney fashion victim ... Michelle, Jacqui, Theresa and Amanda followed the same basic make-up routine but all retained their very individual styles – they still all look like *themselves*, as you can see on pages 48–49.

But what if you want to achieve a more dramatic look – for fancy dress or for a party, whether it's futuristic or retrospective.

On the next four pages we've tried to give you a few ideas. With the first two pictures we picked a very simple classic look and used the same idea on two very different faces. Although each face 'interprets' the look in a completely differ-ent way, it suits them both equally well. For the second two pictures we make no excuses!!! Vicky is *Holly Gram* – a futuristic look from a TV series, where Wendy created a make-up which drew on such far-flung influences as Japanese Kabuki and London punk! As for Sarah – what can we say? Doris Day, eat your heart out! But the influences from the fifties and sixties never seem to date.

Dramatic looks are not as difficult or complicated to put together as you may think. With a few subtle changes to your normal make-up, you can achieve a very different effect – complemented by hairstyles and clothes. It's largely a matter of experimenting and having fun!

By the way, don't think you have to *be* glamorous to end up *looking* glamorous – here we all are BAREFACED – !!!

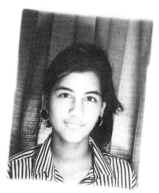
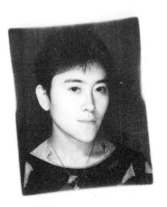
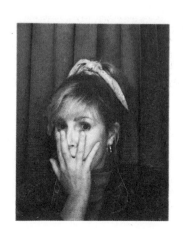
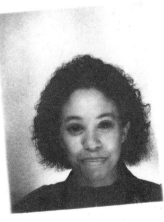

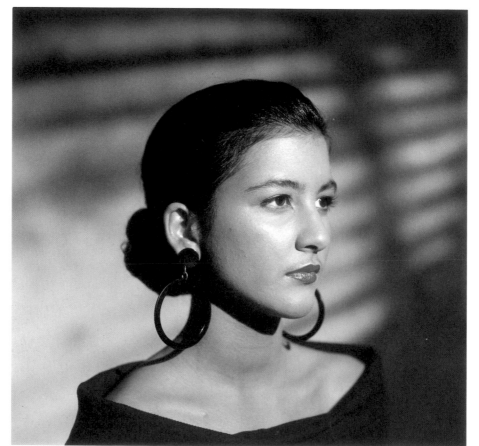

tj

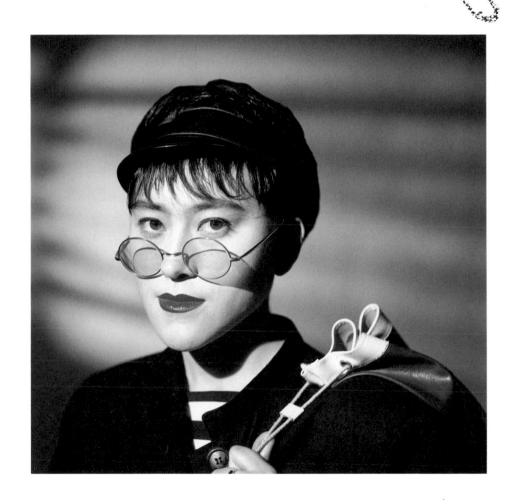

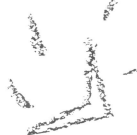

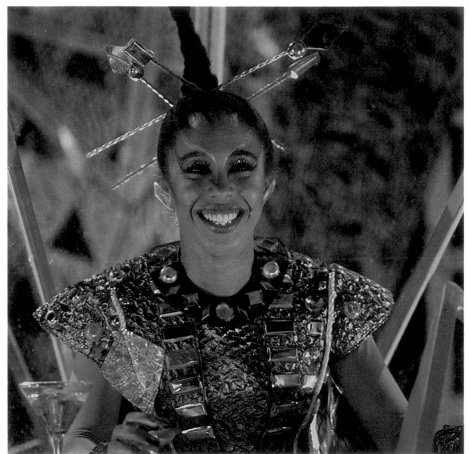

holly gram

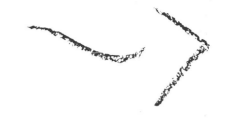

doris

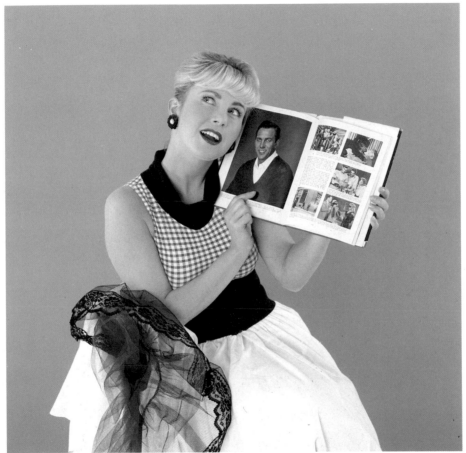

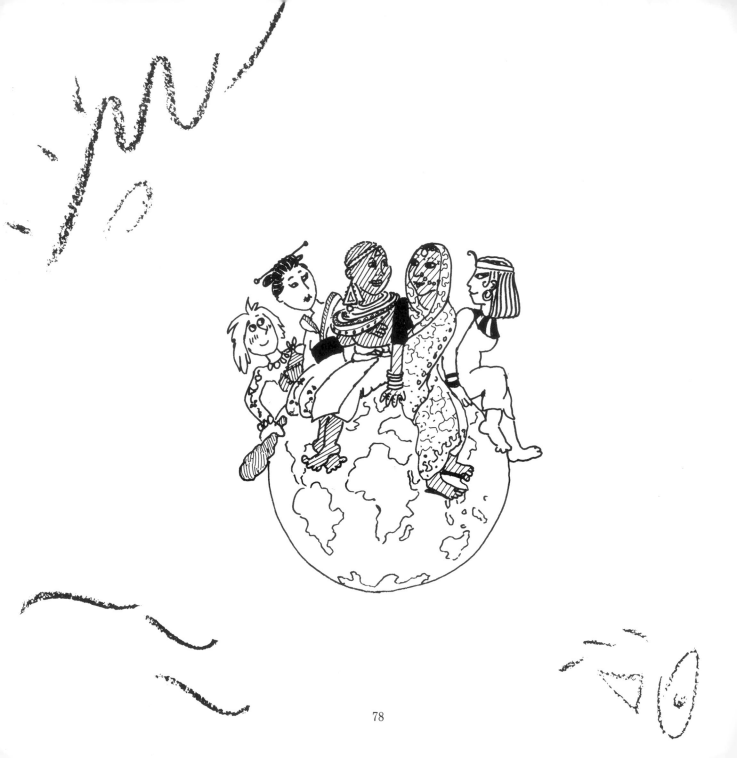

going global

For centuries people all around the world have used paints and dyes to decorate their faces and bodies for both spiritual and purely decorative purposes. Most of us know about the blue body paint called 'woad' used by the Ancient Britons and the distinctive tribal markings of Red Indians, but as recently as the late nineteenth century a standard American book on *male* etiquette advised the use of 'hair dye, paint, face powder and eye shadow.'

So, what's happened since then? Have we become less adventurous? Not really, because the more multi-racial a society we become, the more we feel free to borrow ideas from each other's cultures, as well as from the past. One of the most exciting aspects of living in a multi-cultural society is the way in which ideas can be thrown together. Food and music are obvious examples, fashion of course, and now, make-up.

By combining styles – eastern and western – you can create any number of individual looks . . . whether it's kohl/kajal (from Egypt and India) around your eyes on a very white base – a very Japanese and Chinese ceremonial look – or flashes and dots of bright colour across your face – reminiscent of African tribal decoration.

Coming next are Mimi, Kalpana and Miti to give you an idea of three very different starting points from their own cultures. Then Morwenna sneaks in at the end to steal a bit from each one!

But first, here they are before Wendy got hold of them . . .

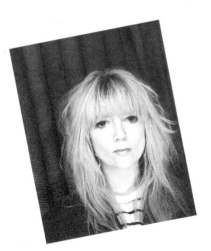
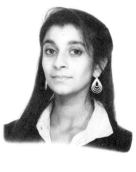
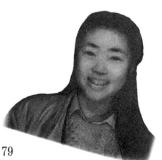
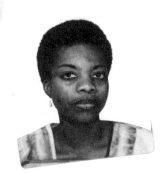

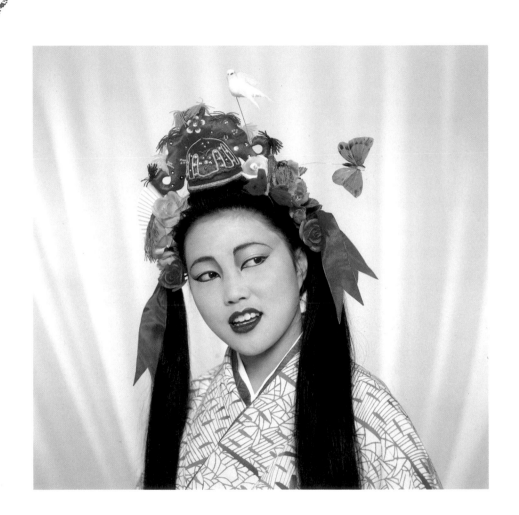

mimi

kalpana

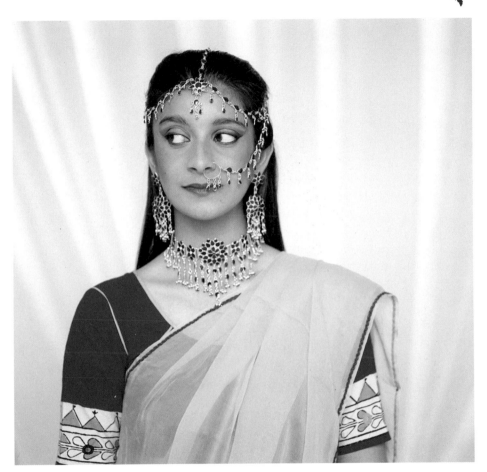

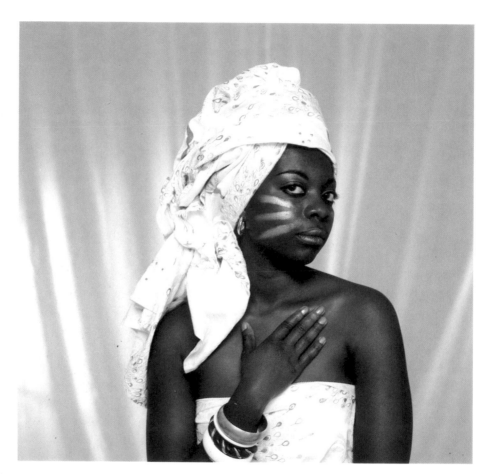

miti

morwenna

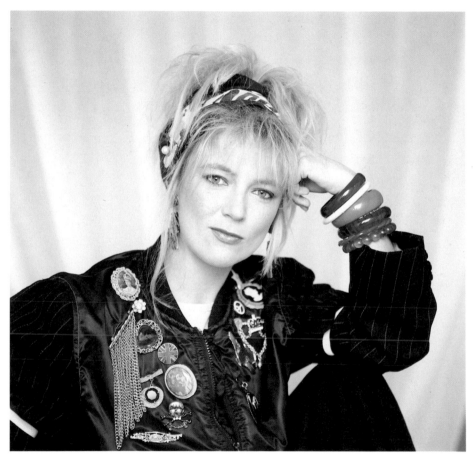

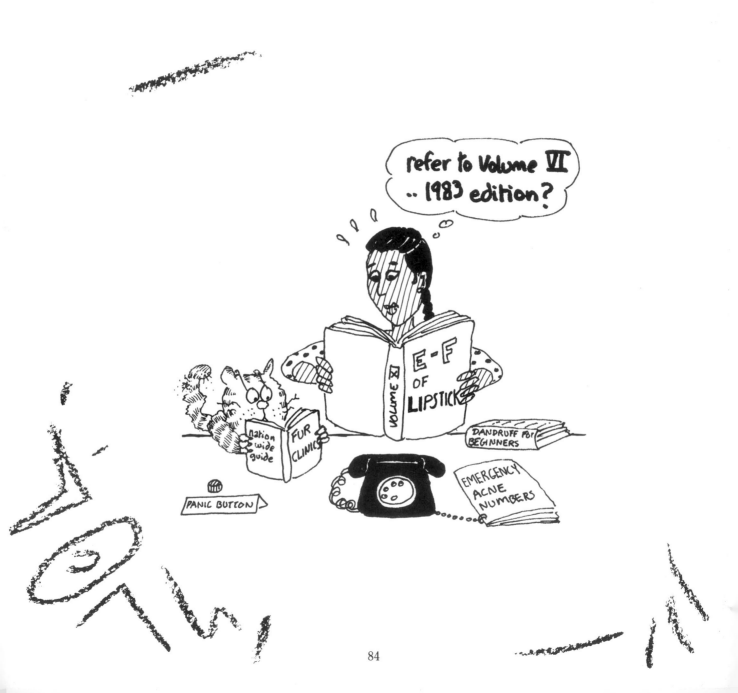

where to find it

- skin care info
- camouflage
- animal testing
- the experts
- useful addresses

AVON
Nunn Mills Road
Northampton
NN1 5PA
064 2324

🐾 Avon cosmetics are sold through representatives who visit your home.

BARRY M
Unit 1 Bittacy Business Park
Bittacy Hill, Mill Hill East
London NW7 1BA
01 349 2992

BEAUTY WITHOUT CRUELTY
37 Avebury Avenue
Tunbridge, Kent
TN9 1TL
Tunbridge 365291

BODY REFORM LTD
Freepost
Bridgend
Mid Glamorgan
CF31 3BR

🐾 With forty of their own shops in the UK, their speciality is using natural products which have not been tested on animals.

BODY SHOP
24 Old Bond St
London W1X 3DA
01 491 7501

CHANEL
76 Jermyn St
London SW1
01 930 1030

COLOURFAST
c/o Max Factor

ESTEE LAUDER
71–72 Grosvenor Street
London W1
01 493 9271

FASHION FAIR
Rubella House
245 Goswell Road
London EC1
01 278 8707

FLORI ROBERTS
158 Notting Hill Gate
London W11 3QG
01 229 4224

🐾 Available from big department stores such as Selfridges and Dickins & Jones in London or by 'Party Girl' representatives who will visit your home.

HELENA RUBINSTEIN
Central Avenue
Poole Road
West Molesley
01 979 7744

LANCOME
14 Grosvenor St
London W1X 0AQ
01 493 6811

LEICHNER
15/18 Hawthorne Road
Eastbourne
0323 641244

MAHOGANY
3 Girton Close
Mildenhall
Suffolk
0638 716962

MARTHA HILL
Freepost
Corby
NN17 3BR
078 085 259

MAXI
c/o Max Factor

	full range of foundation colours	only suitable for european, mediterranean skin	only suitable for darker tones	full skin-care range	on sale in major department stores in U.K.	on sale throughout the U.K. in chemists	on sale throughout U.K. in their own salons	provides trained assistants to stores	offers mail order service	offers separate brushes and accessories
avon		●		●						
barry m	●					●				●
beauty without cruelty		●		●		●			●	●
body reform ltd		●		●			●	●	●	
body shop		●						●	●	●
chanel	●			●	●			●		●
colourfast		●						●		
estee lauder		●		●	●			●	●	
fashion fair	●			●	●				●	●
flori roberts	●		●	●					●	●
helena rubinstein	●				●	●		●	●	
lancome		●		●	●	●		●		
leichner	●			●	●			●		●
mahogany			●	●				●		●
martha hill		●		●					●	
maxi		●			●	●		●		

87

MARY QUANT
75 Davies St
London W1
01 493 7252

MAX FACTOR
Watermans Park, Brentford
Middlesex
TW8 0DS
01 568 4333

MINERS
75 Davies St
London W1
01 493 7252

MOLTON BROWN
– THE COLOUR FREEDOM RANGE
58 South Molton St
London W1Y 1HH
01 499 2046/7

PARADISE COSMETICS
500 Chesham House
150 Regent St
London W1R 5SA
439 6288

PONDS/CUTEX
Cheesborough Ponds Ltd
Victoria Road
London NW10 6NA
07535 57191

RIMMEL
c/o 9 Orme Court
London W2 4RL
01 637 1621

YVES ROCHER
664 Victoria Rd
South Ruislip
Middlesex
HA4 0NY
01 403 4944

Specialise in natural products but only available in four tones, light, medium, dark, ivory.

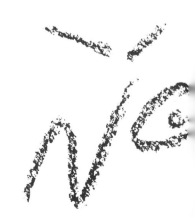

	full range of foundation colours	only suitable for european, mediterranean skin	only suitable for darker skin -ones	full skin-care range	on sale in major department stores in U.K.	on sale throughout the U.K. in chemists	on sale throughout U.K. in their own salons	provides trained assistants to stores	offers mail order service	offers separate brushes and accessories
mary quant		X			X	X		X		
max factor		X		X	X	X		X		
miners		X			X	X		X		
molton brown		X		X				X	X	X
paradise cosmetics			X							
ponds/cutex		X			X	X				
rimmel		X				X		X		
yves rocher		X		X	X			X	X	

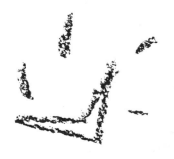

The following companies don't manufacture cosmetics but specialise in skin care ranges using good natural products and also provide excellent skin care advice through their own stores or counters.

Happily most companies no longer feel they need to test their products on animals. For further information:

CLARINS
Metro House
58 St James St
London SW1

CLINIQUE
54 Grosvenor Square
London W1

R.S.P.C.A.
Research Animal Dept
Causeway
Horsham
West Sussex RH12 1HG
0403-64181

Available in most major dept stores and chemists. Trained advice given on their counters in dept stores.

Available from leading chemists and Department stores. They provide fully trained skin care experts for free skin care advice.

CHOOSE CRUELTY FREE
B.U.A.V.
16a Crane Grove
London N7 8LB
01-700-4888

CULPEPPER
Hadstock Road
Linton Cambridge
CB1 6NJ

GERARD
Gerard House
736 Christchurch Road
Bournemouth
Dorset

17 stores in the UK. Send an sae to above address for locations and mail order catalogue.

Skin care products, perfumes and oils based on natural herbs and vitamines. Available from chemists.
For leaflets and details of their mail order service write to above address.

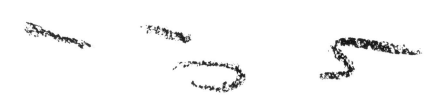

camouflage

We've included this as a separate section as it can be a distressing experience having to deal with birth marks, skin discolorations and scars and yet many of these can be covered up with any one of the many excellent products on the market. Most of them come in a wide range of colours and can be mixed to match your skin tone exactly. Those marked with an asterisk are at present available on doctors prescription.

*COVERMARK: Midex Point
PO Box 25
Arundel, Sussex

*DERMACOLOUR: Charles Fox
22 Tavistock St
London WC2

*KEROMASK: Innoxa UK Ltd
202 Terminus Road
Eastbourne, Sussex

*VEIL: Blare and Co
The Byre House
Nr Masham
N. Yorks HG4 4NF

*BOOTS COVERING CREAM: from the larger branches of Boots

CLINIQUE CONTINUOUS COVERAGE: From Clinique counters

DERMABLEND: From Flori Roberts counters

COMPLETE COVER MAKE UP: Almay counters

CREAM CAMOUFLAGE: Bretlands

PANSTICK & ERACE: Max Factor counters

For further information and a list of trained camouflage volunteers throughout the country contact Rita Roberts, the Red Cross National Headquarters, 9 Grosvenor Crescent, London, SW1X 7EJ.

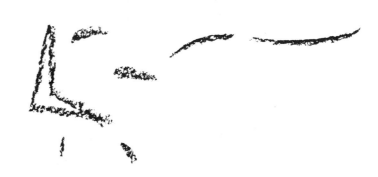

the experts

❧ Here are a few addresses if you fancy coming down to London for the day for a bit of expert advice. Also check your local phone book and newspapers for details in your own area.

THE BEAUTY TRAINING CENTRE
4 Manor Studios
Flood Street
London SW3 5SR

❧ Model Della Finch gives expert classes in make up for darker skins. Courses start at £50 plus VAT.

FACE FACTS
75 George Street
London W1
Tel 01-486-8287

❧ Stephen Glass gives make up lessons. Phone for details.

CHARLES FOX MAKE UP STUDIO
22 Tavistock Street
London WC2 7PY
Tel 01-240 3111

Make up designer Rosemary Swinfield offers a variety of make up lessons ranging from a basic make up lesson for £20 to a bridal or glamour look from £28. Specialities also include camouflage make up and theatrical make up.

FLORI ROBERTS
158 Notting Hill Gate
London W11 3QG
Tel 01-229 4224

People come from all over the world, not only to sample their products, but also to be made up by one of their expert assistants. Their speciality is darker skins. Ring for further details.

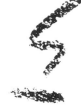

useful addresses

THE HEALTH EDUCATION COUNCIL
78 New Oxford Street
London WC1A 1AH

They offer a large library and resources centre with health care information. Open nine till five Monday to Friday. Send large SAE for free leaflets on health care.

THE ROYAL LONDON
HOMEOPATHIC HOSPITAL
Great Ormond Street
London WC1N 3HR

Write for free advice about homeopathic and natural treatments in your area.

THE MEDICAL ADVISORY SERVICE
10 Barleymow Passage
London W4 49H
Tel 01-994-9874

THE LONDON SKIN HOSPITAL
Lisle Street
London WC2
Tel 01-437-8383

THE NATIONAL EXCEMA SOCIETY
Tavistock Square
London WC1
Tel 01-388-4097

VITILIGO (Skin pigment problems) group.

For information and guidance write to Vitiligo. Audrey Mantle, 79 Old Park Avenue, Enfield, Middlesex.

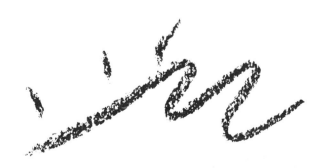

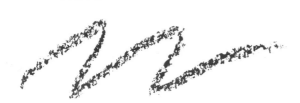

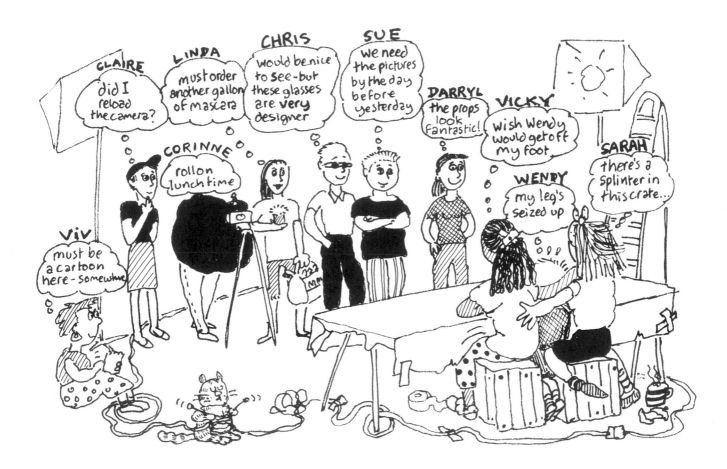

acknowledgements

les girls

Miti Ampona
Morwenna Banks
Mimi Chueng
Mary Hamilton
Tairi Hassen
Theresa Hau
Amanda Hussein
Mo Pickering
Kalpana Shah
Jacqui Tangeney
Michelle Wright

Stylist: Darryl Black
Make Up Artist: Wendy Freeman
Assisted by: Linda Burns
Photographer's Assistant: Claire Pollock

TOGS AND ACCESSORIES SUPPLIED BY
Condor Cycles, Falmers, For Eyes,
Adrian Mann, Monix, Pamplemousse,
Pineapple, Ms. Bones' dress supplied to
Cosmic by Brigitte, Pink Soda, Swatch

MAKE-UP SUPPLIED BY
Lancome, Barry M, Mahogany, Molton
Brown (Colour Freedom Range), Flori
Roberts, Rimmel, Miss Selfridge,
Kirsty Klimo

VERY SPECIAL THANKS TO
Christy Campbell, Douglas da Costa and
Sandra, Todd Edwards, Ann Ferguson of
Which, Harry, Marjie and Laura Greene,
John Henshall for the Holly Gram
picture, Mr and Mrs Licorish, Tony May, Rita
Roberts, Paul Shearer, Mike Smith, Rob
Thomas, The Sylvia Young Theatre School,
Andy Maslen

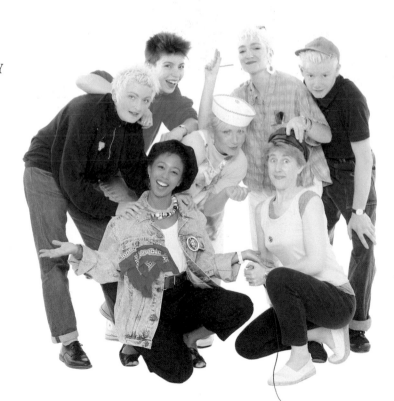

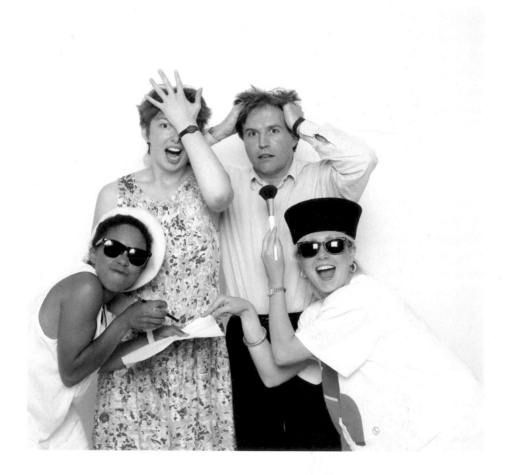

Vicky and Sarah force the editors' hands . . .